Staring Down a Dream

A Mom, a Marathoner, a Mission

Julie B. Hughes

The information quoted, "Adequate carbohydrate intake can safeguard your glycogen storage and protein stores and support blood sugar levels during exercise, helping you sustain energy during your hard workouts and protect your immune system. The research on carbohydrates may look conflicting

Front cover photo: taken by MarathonFoto.

The author has changed some names to protect the privacy of friends and family members mentioned in this book.

All poems were written by the author — Julie B. Hughes

Dedication

For the runner who dreams to race The Boston Marathon. Keep going, keep pushing courage. Never give up! For all the mother runners—Keep pressing on! Dream big—let our child(ren) be the reason to keep lacing up our sneakers. I'll see you on the road.

Contents

Preface

Dear Reader,

I reference 2003 several times in the book because this was the year I was told to stop running. This was the year I was set to run The Boston Marathon yet my pain (emotional and physical) was too great. My body had enough. I needed to listen. I needed to face myself.

As you read my story, there are details that you may be curious about or wonder how I got to this point in my journey. If you want more of a back story of my healing and the many challenges and troubles I faced and overcame, I invite you to read my memoir, My Road—A Runner's Journey Through Persistent Pain to Healing. There are many parts of my narrative that I'm not proud of; however, the exciting piece of my story is God— God is in it.

As I searched for answers, God was there. He placed the right people in my path to guide me, not fix me. No one is here to fix me. A magic pill or quick fix didn't exist— it was an inside job and a turning back to God. He changes everything.

With that said, reading my first book isn't required to understand these pages. However, my readers need to recognize that it was a process to get here and didn't happen overnight. I hope reading my story allows you to face yours with courage and curiosity.

God Bless.

Introduction

You've got to be kidding me. The bus driver is lost?

My mind was racing as I fidgeted in my seat, my legs sticking to the black pigmented leather. I looked down at my watch. We had been on the road for 40 minutes. I was told it would take 30 minutes to get to the start location. *We should already be at the athlete's village getting warmed up and taking in the experience.*

I watched the runners sitting ahead of me, looking around, panicking as they whispered, "This isn't the right way." "We should be here by now." "Oh my gosh, he is lost!"

Oh no! We are lost. I'm not going to get to the start. I am not going to run Boston.

My brain went to the worst-case scenario and my inner judge showed up.

Why did you pick this bus, out of all the buses in line you picked this one. You should've picked a different bus.

GRR, like I was supposed to know the bus driver was going to get lost. I'd been waiting 20 years to run this race, of course, something like this would happen. I was in-between emotions.

Do I cry or laugh?

I looked around at the 48 other runners possibly thinking the same thing. I looked over at my bus buddy and her eyes were closed, resting. She was relaxed. She had no idea what was going on.

Do I tell her? No, we will get there, just be patient, it will be fine.

I took some deep breaths.

Relax, Julie, relax, don't freak out. You will get to the race today. You will be right on time. Ugh, I can't believe this is happening. Here I go again… right back to the negative.

I looked out the window trying to focus on something else — something to shift my mindset.

Look at the trees. Oh yes, the red and orange leaves are gorgeous.

This distracts me for a bit and then we come to a stop.

What's going on?

I craned my head over the seat in front of me and peeked over. Through the bus window, I spotted a police car blocking the road motioning the bus driver to stop. My mind begged for the police officer to let us through.

We're all runners. We need to get to the start. We're late. Please let us through.

A runner stepped off the bus, a perfect time to relieve himself as the policeman approached. I didn't hear much of the conversation other than, "No, I'm sorry. I can't let you through." A few runners ahead of me shouted, "We need to get off this bus." "The cop is not going to let us through." "Do you trust this guy getting us to the start line? He is lost!"

I panicked.

What should I do? I better get off too.

"We can walk and find our way to the start," another runner announced. I stood up to see runners lining up in the aisle waiting to get off.

I better go with them.

I figured it was better to be with a group to find our way. I looked at my bus buddy sitting next to me and told her I was going to walk. She shrugged and moved her legs to the side to let me out. I slipped past her and joined the line of runners making their way off the bus. My stomach flip-flopped at what was occurring. This was not in the plan yet I refused to let this ruin my first Boston Marathon experience. I would get to the start line.

Do not panic, breathe and relax, you are not alone.

Chapter One
The Medal

Ready to fly
A bird soaring high
Forward motion, beats
the commotion. Fresh air
even if it's cold.
I am bold.

The yellow and blue box arrived at my front door—FIN-ISHER was scrolled in bold letters across the top.

YES! The unicorn medal is here.

I did a happy dance carrying the box inside. I tore off the tape, untucked the side flaps, and opened the box. The unicorn medal was displayed in the center. I sat down and stared at it before gently picking it up. I was thrilled to see the silver unicorn with 2020 in yellow print at the bottom of the medal. The year of quarantine may have distorted a few things for me but this medal in my hands was real and true, the silver lining.

I slipped the medal over my head. The blue-yellow satin ribbon was soft against the back of my neck. I couldn't wait to show my family. Brindsley and Delaney were at school. Jeff was at work. I celebrated anyway. I thanked my body and mind for another finish. My first Boston Marathon medal.

I did it!

I walked around the house with a big grin looking down every few seconds to check it out. I was over the moon until my inner judge, Aunt Phoebe spoke up.

Does this really count? Your dream was to run the Boston Marathon but you didn't really run it. You weren't there. You weren't in Boston.

The grin turned to a grimace as I sat back down taking the medal off my neck. I placed it back into the box.

Sigh…this is true.

I didn't go to Boston and run the course. I didn't experience the Scream Tunnel or the famous Heartbreak Hill. I didn't run the streets like Kathrine Switzer, Bobbi Gibb, or the many other brave women before me. My dream wasn't complete. I stared at the medal in the box wanting to celebrate yet my thoughts were defeated.

My dream was half-achieved in my mind. I received the bib number, shirt, and medal in the mail yet I didn't run the Boston Marathon course. The Boston Marathon was moved to a virtual race due to the COVID-19 pandemic. It meant I would run the 26.2 miles on roads or trails of my choosing. The course would be up to me. There would be no traveling to Boston. There would be no Scream Tunnel or Heartbreak Hill. There would be no crowds, volunteers to block the roads, cowbells ringing, or cheers from spectators.

I did try to make it more than just any long run. I recruited my family for hydration stops, friends to cheer me on, and my children to hold the finishing tape. It was a wonderful experience, don't get me wrong, I was grateful. Yet, as I sat at my kitchen table I didn't feel settled. My dream didn't feel achieved, and I knew it wouldn't until I got to Boston.

I made up my mind that I would keep training with my intention to race The Boston Marathon in 2021. Luckily, my family was supportive and Jeff knew how important this was to me. He's known about it since we met in 2011. It was my mission to get there, and I kept my faith that it would be so.

I had no control over whether Boston would hold the in-person marathon next year or if it would be virtual again. Yet, what I could control was my attitude, how I showed up, and how I managed my mind about it all. I kept an optimistic mindset and I prayed. Deep down I was certain things would turn around and road races would be held again. The story I told myself and believed was I would run The Boston Marathon next year in Boston. It was better than the alternative and energized me heading into the new year.

I connected with my performance coach, Joel Sattgast, PT, DPT. We had been working together since 2018. His coaching style, knowledge, and guidance were a big reason I am running strong and healthy today. He was a great coach but more importantly a great person and friend. He had come alongside me through my setbacks and health challenges in a big way, and to have him in my corner was a blessing.

He had not only prepared me physically for the marathon distance but he also prepared me mentally. His encouragement to practice mantras, or thoughts that would keep me going when the going got tough, and visualizations were important tools for my performance. I told him my sights were back on racing The Boston Marathon. *I want to run the course.* He was excited to hear I wanted to keep going and was on board for another year of coaching. I was thrilled. He was optimistic that the marathon would take place in Boston. Joel had a great attitude and mindset, another reason why I loved working with him. It rubbed off on me, and I wanted to show up the same way.

Chapter Two
I'm In

Lace-up your sneakers
No responsibility
You and the road, free

It's early but I love the quiet morning runs. I get to greet the morning and set my intention for the day. The roads are dark on Watervale Road until I make it into the village. My runs are in this direction—out of the darkness and into the light. The street lights guide my way along with the moon as I enter the village.

I make a turn to the left where I head up the sidewalk past the swan pond. Two beautiful white swans are curled up in the water. I slow down to take a look wondering if they are sleeping. At that moment, one gracefully lifts her long neck almost as if she heard my thought.

Good morning beautiful swan.

I pick up my pace and smile at the morning. I'm so lucky to live in Manlius, New York where I get to see two swans on my morning runs. I'm so glad we moved here even during the pandemic and crazy house market. It was just after the

Boston virtual marathon in September 2020 when we started packing up to make our move across town.

We made the right decision. I love the hilly country roads—the perfect training ground for The Boston Marathon. I had no idea if it would happen this year— yet I kept telling myself it would. I kept the faith that 2021 would be the year for me—the year that I would travel to Boston and race the marathon. I was waiting for the email to show up in my inbox—the one that reads, the 125th Boston Marathon is a go and you are in. Until then, I would stay optimistic and stick to my training plan.

I trained through the week on my own and looked forward to Saturdays when I met up with my run buddy, Felicia, for our long run. We knew hills would be important in our training and we didn't need to go far —Manlius, New York was surrounded by hills, rolling terrain, and climbing elevations. I was excited to train locally and just step right out my door. The hilly country roads were breathtaking and peaceful. It was a challenge we embraced and looked forward to. These hills and these roads would prepare me for The Boston Marathon.

***

I was getting anxious to know if the marathon was going to be held or if it would be another virtual event. It was mid-March when I got an email that read:

Dear Boston Marathoner,

We write to share with you that the Boston Athletic Association has announced if road races are allowed to take place as part of the Massachusetts reopening plan, the 125th Boston Marathon on Monday, October 11, 2021, will feature a field size of 20,000 entrants. Registration for the in-person Boston Marathon will take place the week of April 20-23, 2021.

The Boston Athletic Association will celebrate the milestone 125th running of the Boston Marathon both as an in-person race (Monday, October 11) and a virtual race (October 8-10).

Sincerely,
The Boston Athletic Association

I was relieved that it was a possibility. There was a plan and a date. I marked my calendar for April 20th to register at 10 a.m. I would use my qualifying time from The Wineglass Marathon in 2018. I was grateful this was an option as most of the 2020 race schedule had been canceled. I needed to meet the time standards for my age group (40-44) and gender to be considered for acceptance. I acknowledged that instead of 30,000 entrants, they were accepting 20,000. I was hopeful that my time was fast enough to make it in.

I prayed that the live marathon would take place even though COVID-19 was still causing a lot of distress and uncertainty around the world. New variants were emerging and that was creating some anxiety.

Would this prevent the Boston Marathon from taking place?

It was May 4th, 2021 when I got the news. I was standing in the kitchen, thinking about dinner, when my mind wandered off.

Check your email, maybe there will be something about Boston.

My laptop was conveniently sitting on the kitchen island calling me to open it. I went straight to my email inbox. In bold letters was the subject—125th Boston Marathon Confirmation of Acceptance—my eyes widened. I clicked on the email to read:

> Dear Julie Hughes,
>
> Congratulations! Your entry into the in-person 125th Boston Marathon on Monday, October 11, 2021, has been accepted.

I let out a shout. My hand covered my mouth in disbelief as I whispered,

Oh my gosh, it's finally going to happen. I'm going to Boston.

I stood in the kitchen staring at the words "congratulations" and "accepted." My voice stuck in my throat. I kept my eyes on the screen as I read it a few more times making sure it was true.

My children were running around the house. Jeff was getting the grill going for dinner. My voice came back in a boom—"I got into Boston! Oh my gosh! We are going to Boston!" Jeff came over to where I stood. I pointed to the computer screen.

He looked at the email with me and hugged me. "That's awesome honey!" The kids heard my shouts and came into the kitchen. I hugged them. We began jumping up and down. They were laughing at my excitement yet they also knew how much this meant to me. The possibility of Boston was now in full view.

The mindset of "I will get there, be patient, and it will happen," paid off. A dream I'd been staring down for two decades was finally going to be celebrated! It was going to happen this time. I could feel it in my bones. Thank you, Lord.

I sent text messages to family and friends who knew how important this goal was to me. I also let my coach know.

We were going to Boston! Let the planning and training truly begin.

Chapter Three
Morning Runner

Long run Saturday
Morning runaway
Legs charge down the road
Self-care to unload
Empty the thoughts with every stride
God will take them captive— your guide
Trust Him in all you do
The spirit lives inside of you
Breathe in love
Exhale fear
Your faith is the anchor
You will make it my dear

At 4:30 a.m. the alarm went off. I had a 40-minute easy run planned. The day was scheduled with no wiggle room. This was the time to run. I laid under the covers wondering if I could change my schedule somehow. My warm blanket made it hard to roll out of bed. I wanted to go back to sleep.

Julie, get up and go! Your clothes are ready for you and the coffee will be brewed when you get back.

Okay, Okay.

I rolled out of bed and dragged myself to the bathroom. I turned the faucet on splashing cold water over my face.

Wake up Julie, you can do this, you will feel better once you get outside. Maybe the stars or moon will be out.

I pulled my shirt over my head and thought about the other runners who were getting up early too. This thought encouraged me as I headed to the door to get my sneakers on. I double-laced my shoes, covered myself in lights and reflective gear, and reached for the doorknob when the question came—*Why do I want to run Boston?*

For me, it took some thought to find the reason. It was part of my mental training that had changed over the years. It kept me focused. Kept me showing up when my brain shouted, *Go back to sleep. Give up on your dream. It's never going to happen. You can run another day.*

Not all mornings did I jump out of bed ready to go—I'm human after all— but when those mornings came I was ready—running clothes laid out with sneakers and a reflective vest at the door. Coffee was set to brew at 5:30 a.m., accountability (*I told my husband I will be back from my run to see him before he leaves for work*) and to find the "why" in it all were some strategies to help me, especially in the fall and winter months.

Why did I get up to run alone in the dark and cold? Why was this goal so important to me? Why did I need to run The Boston Marathon? I've asked these questions many times since 2003. That was my year to race and achieve my dream. Yet, that was the year everything fell apart. The pain took charge of my life. My morning ritual of running was gone and this increased my pain, depression, and self-doubt. Training for marathons was no longer a part of my life—The Boston Marathon was in the backseat—though my dream never extinguished.

During that season of challenge, my dream never died. It stayed with me like a good friend. When I made my way out of the darkness, my dream to run The Boston Marathon was the light at the end of the tunnel. I believed my dream kept me moving through the dark seasons. It gave me something to fight for and changed me. So I ask myself these questions again at 4:30 a.m. as I grab the doorknob. *Why do I want to run Boston? Why am I still pursuing this dream? Why wasn't running the virtual Boston Marathon enough?*

I knew why. I wanted to experience it myself. I wanted to see the crowds of spectators filling the roads cheering and holding signs. I wanted to hear what it's like to run through the Scream Tunnel. I wanted to feel the climb of Heartbreak Hill and the victory of crossing the finish line. I had read about it all yet I wanted my own experience.

Even after I finished the virtual Boston Marathon it wasn't enough. I got the medal and the jacket. It was my first. Yet, my dream was not complete, and I knew it wouldn't be until I ran the roads from Hopkinton to Boston like the women before me.

I wanted to run this for my friends who died wanting to run it but never did. Now that I was a mom, I had taught my children to keep chasing their dreams no matter how long it may take to reach them. I had many reasons to get out of bed and train for this marathon. It's why this dream meant so much to me.

***

My morning ritual had included running, but since 2020, I added in writing. I would run and then sit down to write with a hot cup of coffee. I'd found my creative juices flowed best just after a run. My notebook was ready for me to jot down ideas for poems or stories. The road brought back memories—a smell, a sight, or even a song that could take me back in time without a warning. It happened to me on one particular run.

I was thinking about what to have for breakfast as I pumped my arms and legs down the country road when the smell of cow manure filled my nostrils. The distinct odor sent me back to my childhood on the dairy farm. My memory took a u-turn back in time and gave me something to write about when I got home.

I wrote down memories to heal, process, and let go. I felt free. I felt lighter. It was another tool to keep me moving forward—to not get stuck in the past. I found writing to be very similar to running. One word after another, one foot in front of the other—Go, Go, Go! A solitary practice that felt like I had company, encouragement, and support. "Run to write" was my mantra. On some days, when I didn't want to get out of bed, writing was my motivation to get going. What would I see? What would I hear? What would God place on my heart? What would spark my writing for today? I knew I had to get out and run. I was grateful running gave me an outlet to find the words. Just when I thought I would run out of words, they hovered on the clouds, swayed on the trees, or floated with the breeze for me to catch and jot down. This was when I felt closer to God, and He gave me the words to write.

I flashed and glowed down the road. I saw a cloud form out of my mouth with each stride. I watched it circle and then disappear. Another one escaped me as I bound down the road. I pulled my hat over my ears. The cars and trucks passed by, seemingly to be in a hurry. *Where were they going?* I stayed focused and alert. I concentrated on the morning, and on my surroundings. *What do I see? What do I hear?* Curiosity grows on the road. Where is the bunny going? Look at all those whitetail deer, wow, do you hear the birdsong? Look at the moon, guiding me, my run buddy for the morning.

The road to the village was dark with minimal street lights. Fall was here and change was in the air. The children were back to school and Boston was less than a month away. My inner judge, Aunt Phoebe, squeaked in, "Are you good enough to run Boston? Are you sure you're ready? I don't think you've done enough hills." I know she was just looking out for me yet I wished she wouldn't. She was a wicked witch that lives inside my mind. I would have loved to wave a magic wand over myself, particularly my brain, so I never had to hear her again. Her judgment, her fear, and her self-doubt are a daily commentary I'm sure I wouldn't miss, yet I'm human. I accepted she will show up, and when she does, I get to decide what to do next. Listen and believe everything she says or listen and challenge her with a question. *What else could be true? Is this thought serving me?*

Curiosity was the key for me. I found myself living with more energy, joy, and peace, and that was a gift from God. *If I could acknowledge the sentence or thought that wasn't serving me well or wasn't true then I could take power back. The truth would set me free. I could tell Aunt Phoebe (my inner judge) to let go of the fear or the anxiety. I did have a magic wand if I chose the mindset of curiosity and to not give the enemy a seat at the table.*

***

One training run I had was an hour-fartlek — an intermix of fast running with periods of slower running. *Isn't fartlek a funny name? Who even came up with that word? (I'll research it later.)* I couldn't wait to tell my children when I got home as I smiled to myself. I grabbed my hydration vest and placed two soft flasks in the front pockets. My coach had encouraged me to practice taking in fluids for all runs over an hour. I had this vest for four years now and it was still in great shape. It has been a welcome addition to my training gear.

During marathon races, the vest allowed me to carry my nutrition without slowing down or stopping at the on-course stations. I used to wear a waistband with bottles attached but had a hard time finding the best fit or keeping it from bouncing around as I ran. I remember past races having to adjust, re-velcro, or frequently reposition the band around my waist as I was running. It was very frustrating and slowed me down so you can imagine my relief when I purchased a vest. The vest was snug without bouncing or chafing which was a huge benefit when running longer distances. I placed it over my clothes, snapped it in the front, and off I went— no fidgeting with it while I ran. It was something I depended on like my running sneakers and had allowed me to improve my nutrition timing for race day. I didn't dread wearing it like I did the waistband.

I looked down at my watch—*time to pick up the pace*. I took a few sips from my water flask and then increased my cadence. *Playing with speed today as I alternate my pace from easy to hard, that's a fartlek.* I enjoyed these training sessions—it was fun to switch up the pace and it kept me focused mentally. The run seemed to fly by— an hour had already passed.

I slid open the door, sweat dripping from my face, Brindsley and Delaney were at the breakfast table. They were already eating. I was so happy to see them and started to smile as the word fartlek came to mind.

"Hey mama, how was your run?" Brindsley asked between spoonfuls of granola. Delaney looked up from her bowl.

"It was great! I did a fartlek today." I managed to keep a straight face.

They both stopped eating and exploded with laughter. I was pretty sure all they heard was the word fart!

"Mom, you said fart!" They both said in unison.

Yup, I was right. I began to laugh too. I guess that was all I heard as well, and laughed with them as I grabbed a cup of coffee.

Oh, how I love that my children laughed at that silly word. This is what I love most about motherhood, the laughter. Isn't it the best sound? They always find something to laugh about and that makes me so happy. It helps me lighten up. I can be so serious and stiff—more laughter is what I need these days. I'm still laughing now as I write this and am grateful for the word fartlek, as odd as that sounds. When I'm having a tough day or getting all bent out of shape, I'll just say the word fartlek in front of my kids or to myself. It's better than cursing.

Fartlek…say that out loud a few times today if you need a laugh. I hope it lightens up your mood a bit too. Go ahead — give it a go.

Chapter Four
Marathon Mom

The weather changes
Keep showing up on the road
Lean forward, lean in
You will make it mom
The climb is sometimes long — yet
You have what it takes

"Okay, kids, I'm going to be gone for a few hours each Saturday morning to run."

Brindsley grinned, then shrugged. I wondered what he was thinking. I was sure he was shouting, "Yes, mom will be gone, we can watch all the TV we want!"

Delaney looked concerned, "When will you be home?"

"I'll be home after you eat breakfast."

"Okay." She stuck her head back in her book. Brindsley went back to playing with his Legos.

This dream came with being clear on my priorities and commitment to my training. The weekends were dedicated to long runs, meal planning, and recovery. I limited my social engagements during the week and weekends to make sure I got enough sleep though this was easier with COVID-19 still hanging around. Early bedtime meant less time with Jeff in the evenings.

On Saturday mornings, I would get up early for my long run. Jeff would be home with Brindsley and Delaney and it became their time together to hang out with dad and watch a TV show. I could imagine their conversation going something like this in the early hours.

"Where is mama? I'm hungry."

"She's out for a run."

"Oh, yeah, she's training for the Boston Marathon. She gets up so early. Hey, Dad, let's watch TV since mom isn't here."

"I thought you were hungry."

"No, let's watch TV instead."

I was grateful my children were at this age. I did miss them not needing me as much yet I was glad to be in this season of parenting. It certainly wasn't easy at any age, in my opinion. Jeff was supportive of my training and had no problem with me going every Saturday morning. It was his time with the kids; they enjoyed watching TV shows together. He was more than capable of making them breakfast and getting them what they needed, yet a piece of me felt I needed to be the one. I needed to be available and around to help them.

I couldn't be gone too long. *Is this the mother's guilt or my need to control and feel wanted?* Or maybe it was that I didn't want to miss out on something. I wasn't certain. Yet, the mom guilt liked to show up often. *Oh! Look who it is—Aunt Phoebe convincing me that I'm a terrible mom because I'm out for a run and chasing a dream.* She liked to make me feel bad for taking care of myself. I laughed at her. I knew her tricks and it wouldn't work this time.

Yes, I was spending hours on the road away from my children yet it was my time for me. I had a friend say to me once, "Self-care is so important because then we can be our best for others." I truly believed this. I was at my best for my family when I ran, took care of myself, and had a goal to achieve.

They knew they were loved, and I believed that I was teaching them through my actions. Yes, self-care, movement, eating healthy balanced meals, and setting goals were important. And discipline, dedication, persistence, and courage too. I prayed this was what they were learning through my actions.

***

One morning after a run, I stood in the bathroom with my kids as we all got ready for the day. They were washing their faces and I seemed to think I needed to micromanage what was going on. *Don't forget your nose, make sure you floss, and brush your teeth.* I looked down at my bare feet. I crinkled my nose. My toenails were pretty beaten up from running.

I laughed in disgust, "My toenails are still purple." I didn't mean to say it out loud.

Delaney looked over at me and smiled, "Mom, you are unique."

I nodded my head and grinned, "What a beautiful thing to say, Delaney. Yes, I think you are right, I am unique. Thank you."

My inner judge, Aunt Phoebe, was ready to launch in. *Your toenails are disgusting. You better get some socks on.* Yet Delaney's comment shut her down. My thoughts were full of gratitude towards my daughter and my running feet.

Thank you feet for the miles we continue to run.

Let's give ourselves permission to celebrate our uniqueness... purple toenails and all!

***

What did it take to train for a marathon? If you answered prioritizing sleep, nutrition, mindset, strength training, and running you were correct. Yet, if you're a mother like me, add in grace, the "lighten up" wand, and laughter. I learned very quickly that I would need to let some things go—dishes in the sink, laundry piled high, messy rooms—traded for more sleep, meal planning, and time in the kitchen cooking meals. I relied on laughter when I felt overwhelmed by the day-to-day responsibilities trying to get the best of me.

It's okay to have dishes in the sink. It's okay to finish the laundry over the weekend. These gentle reminders helped me let go of my desire for perfection. When I felt my body start to tense up or my breathing shallow, lighten up and laughter were my two intentions for the day. My children were a blessing to help me practice these intentions.

My son Brindsley tells me I boss him around. *Sigh...I like to think I'm gently reminding him.* One night I recalled him not getting into the shower when I asked. I decided to set a timer, "Brindsley ten more minutes then it's time for a shower, reading, then bed." When the time was up, he was sneaking around the house hiding from me. *Oh geez, not again!*

"Okay, Brindsley, time for a shower" in my most calm and cheery voice.

If I didn't prompt him, would he even clean himself up? My guess was no. Anyways, he knew the routine at eight years old, yet I found myself reminding him. Every night was the same, shower, brush, floss, mouth rinse, yada yada. This night was no different so I thought...

Brindsley shouted, "Mom you are a bath boss!"

GRRR. Did he just call me a bath boss?

I laughed out loud at those words and I couldn't stop. My laugh was loud and tears welled up in my eyes—a true belly laugh. I was not sure that was the reaction he wanted or expected as he ran to his room and shut the door. Yet I was giving myself a high-five! I laughed instead of getting my panties in a bunch and that was something to celebrate.

Why am I telling you this story? Because during your training you may need to find the things, the small things to celebrate. Training can be long especially when the seasons change. Motherhood and training can be challenging so I encourage you to find moments to laugh, have fun, and enjoy the chaos a bit. I've learned to be more flexible, pivot, and adapt on the fly—motherhood has given me these skills. I'm noticing this has helped with my marathon training and when things come up that I don't plan or anticipate.

For instance, when I got an email from The Boston Athletic Association two weeks before the marathon regarding what's allowed and what's prohibited on race day. I began reading, and, at first, everything was pretty standard until I read that running vests were prohibited. *What?!* I had no idea. This was what I'd been training with for the last five years. I'd worn the vest for all the other marathons I had raced in. I used two soft flasks, put them in the front pockets, and put my energy gels in the side pockets. I didn't think this would be a problem for Boston. I was wrong. *Of course, running vests would be prohibited, Julie!* I was ashamed that the bombing in 2013 slipped my mind. *Why didn't you think about that? How could you forget?* I tended to beat myself up. There I go.

My mind started to spiral. *What am I going to do? How will I carry my hydration? I haven't practiced with anything else.* The questions were racing. I scrambled to think about what I would do if I didn't carry my hydration. I texted my coach to see what his thoughts were and if he knew of any other options. I also let him know about the email to make sure I was reading it right. He gathered the same conclusion from the wording of the email—a running vest isn't allowed. He sent me back a text with a link to buy a running waistband to carry hydration—this was the band he used to run with. I was relieved. I let out a breath. My shoulders came down from my ears as I clicked on the link to order. I purchased two different sizes to make sure I got the right fit—nothing worse than hydration bottles bouncing around as you run. I paid extra for overnight shipping so I would have time to practice with it before leaving for Boston. I was hoping it wouldn't jiggle and slide around my waist.

Sigh—this was not the plan. Yet wasn't this life? We think we got it all figured out, plan in place, and then boom. I was reminded I was not in control and to roll with it. I would learn something from this. Maybe the waistband was better than the vest. I would see. For now, I needed to stay calm, pivot, and adapt to this new circumstance. I was grateful Joel knew exactly where to guide me and he kept me calm. What a blessing I had him in my corner.

I scanned the order information and it said I would be getting the running waistbands the next day. I prayed this waistband was the answer to my problem. It said it held two soft flasks in the back pocket and I hoped that was true. It would be frustrating if I couldn't carry my hydration in the early miles of the marathon. I didn't want to get stuck behind other runners at the hydration stops.

I glanced at the clock, 8 p.m., and still no package. No running waistbands. *UGH.* I guess next-day delivery doesn't always mean the next day. The pandemic had caused all sorts of delays in the shipping and delivery of items. *It would come tomorrow—stay patient,* I repeated to myself. I would still have a few days to run with it on and to see which one fit the best.

The next day I saw the package set up against the front door. I was thrilled. They were here! I'd never been so happy to receive a package. I opened both sizes to see which one would fit better. One size was too loose, but the other one fit perfectly. I was so glad I ordered the right size. It held all the hydration and nutrition that I would carry on race day. It fit great around my waist with no bouncing as I gave it a try on my run. Victory! The running waistband was the solution—bump in the road—figured out. Onward!

Chapter Five
Thinner Does NOT Mean Faster

I ignored my body
for a number.
A number on the scale
Is that all I am?
If I just reach that number
Life will change
I will be happy
I will be loved
I will be a faster runner
Yet—
The number never came
The scale cold under my feet
Head down shoulders slouched
in defeat.
I got mad at my body
Consumed by food—
preoccupied with
body image.
Fast runners are thin and lean
that's what they all said.
I heard I was neither—
Is this all I am?

Fat, muscle,
skin, bones.
No— Focus on how you feel,
and what your body can do
instead of what it looks like.
She spoke to me
over the phone
Get to know your body.
Do you feel strong, resilient, and healthy?
What?
A number consumed my mind
that would never allow
me to answer this question.
Would I consider it?
Let the number go
Throw away the scale
Get to know my body
as a beloved friend— Yes
And it's made all the difference.

Food and I hadn't been the best of friends. I had a very poor relationship since childhood. The old story of "thinner meant faster" or "thinner meant better" was a belief I held onto for many years. This was my default story and it led to many years of pain, fatigue, and unhappiness. I truly believed that I wouldn't have gotten this far or be where I am today if I didn't do the hard work to change my mindset around food or had the help to do it.

I was having increased irritable bowel syndrome and stomach pain. It was not only affecting my training but my eating.

What was going on? Was it something I was eating?

I was getting very frustrated. I was finally back to the marathon distance and my stomach pain was here again.

I just won't eat for a few days to calm things down.

Well, how will you train Julie without eating anything? You are ridiculous, that isn't the answer.

I was beating myself up and my inner dialogue was not helpful. My relationship with food needed to change. I'd ignored this part of my story for a long time. I was hoping it would just go away—just shoving it down so it didn't come up was my old strategy. I was fooling myself. I didn't have an issue with food. I was fine. I didn't need help. I would be okay. Deep down I knew I wouldn't. Now as a mother I wanted to let this belief go. This wasn't true or helpful. I found myself slipping back into old thought patterns. I needed help. I was ready to own this part of my story and face myself.

***

I had this fear of getting fat and my unhealthy relationship with food was once again rearing its ugly head. Just when I thought I was good, I would have a setback and it would bring this story to the surface. I would shove it down, ignore it, and move on. This time, I didn't want to do that. I needed to confront my story around my rules about food. These rules were rules I carried around and they were exhausting. *Pay attention to how many calories I consumed each day. Don't eat fat. Avoid too many carbohydrates. Have one dessert a week. And exercise each day to earn what I eat.*

I wanted to enjoy the food and eat it. I didn't want it consuming my thoughts all the time. It was stealing the joy from my training. It was stealing the joy from my life.

When I linked up with Marni Sumbal, MS, RD, CSSD, LD/N, owner of Trimarni Coaching and Nutrition, she permitted me to let go of the food rules. She said I could unlearn them with hard work. I desperately needed to hear this. I was ready to do the work. Her words were even more powerful to me because she was a female endurance athlete. I was eager to start.

She asked if I had any issues now or in the past with an eating disorder. I said no. I lied to her over the phone.

Was I still in denial about that part of my story?

I didn't want to talk about it again, and I certainly didn't want to play the victim. It came out so fast that I was shocked. I was tired of that part of me and just wanted to forget that it ever happened. I didn't have a disorder now so I said no. Yet, I didn't have a healthy relationship with food and I wanted to. I wanted to learn how to fuel myself to improve my performance and figure out whether my stomach pain was something I was eating or not eating.

I wanted to backtrack.

Wait a minute. Yes, I did have an eating disorder for over a decade but I figured it was too late so I didn't mention it.

Her voice was encouraging and calm. I was eager to learn from her about what I could do to change how I was feeling and help my performance. I mentioned I wanted a healthy relationship with food and I hoped this was my way back to it.

She asked, "What are you struggling with and what is your training like?" I wanted her to know that I did have difficulty figuring out how to fuel myself properly for training. I was struggling with body image, what foods to eat, and how much. I shared with her I was training for a marathon.

Marni wanted me to write down what I ate for a few days so she could take a look and get a snapshot of my typical eating. This made me cringe a bit.

Do I have to? How else would she be able to help me without seeing what I was currently eating?

I agreed to write down what I ate for breakfast, lunch, and dinner plus any snacks. She sent me a log to complete. I would then send it back to her via email.

I took a look at the document. She wanted me to write down what I ate before and after runs. She also wanted me to identify where I was eating—in the car, on the go, at the kitchen table. I was also to include what my mood or energy level was when I ate.

I thought these questions were interesting because I had never paid attention to them. In the past, eating was my go-to when I didn't want to feel anything. Yet, I didn't correlate it to my mood or energy level.

I started recording my first day. Breakfast was easy—a chocolate protein shake with one banana and a cup of almond milk. I recorded where I ate—standing at the kitchen counter. I recorded my mood—energized after my run. I continued journaling in my food diary for the next few days.

I wanted to feel better and improve my meal-planning skills. I wanted to pass this on to my children which was a big motivator for me. I wanted this to be a lifestyle—a habit to stay consistent with over the long haul. I didn't want food to consume my thoughts and my day. I was grateful for Marni who was so knowledgeable, and willing to help me. I was like a sponge taking in all she had to say.

She spoke of the daily diet and how important it was to plan balanced meals that included specific amounts of carbohydrates, fat, and protein to keep my body in good health. She reminded me, "The daily diet is the foundation with which your body performs." I was eager to learn how to improve.

I found myself at times skipping lunch. I knew this wasn't ideal or sustainable but I didn't think it was a contributor to my stomach pain.

For the next few days, I was mindful of what I ate and how much. I logged each meal on the sheet and took a deep breath.

Julie, you can do this.

I sent it to Marni and waited to hear from her. I was anxious.

What would she think about my eating habits? Maybe I'm eating too much? What would she think of me?

I wonder what she would say when she saw what I wrote down. I was worried. I was in my head way too much. I reminded myself that she was here to help me. It was okay.

As I stared at my daily logs, I knew I wasn't eating enough. I knew I had some hard work to do around my relationship with food.

Julie keep pushing courage and remember your why.

I was working hard at talking kinder to myself too.

Marni reached out to me the next day, and we scheduled our next session over the phone. She was so encouraging and supportive that I was able to let my worries and anxieties go. Marni made some great suggestions on how to move forward. "I would like you to stop buying the meal replacement shake." I was quiet for a moment and she continued, "Use that money to go get a massage." I nodded as I held the phone to my ear. The replacement shake was a pricey powder that I was buying every month. A massage was a great idea. I was surprised by my eagerness and agreement to let the shake go. I'd been drinking that shake every morning for over three years.

The shake was easy. I didn't have to think. She realized this and encouraged me to eat real food instead. "Okay, I will stop buying the shake," I hesitated. She offered suggestions for morning meals and sent me some handouts with options as well. I liked this and it gave me a resolution. I understood in just two sessions of talking to her that my daily diet needed more balance and she was going to help me. I was going to get better.

She pointed out where I was missing carbohydrates, protein, or fat. She coached me on ways to make more balanced meals in a kind and gentle way. I was catching on and began to plan my meals for the week. I took the time to pay attention to my mood and energy level throughout the day so I could record that on the sheet. I was gaining confidence and Marni was there to check in each week. She helped me add to my fueling needs based on my training. We then talked about fueling before and after runs. "I want you to eat something before every single workout." She suggested taking in some food around 100 calories, 30 minutes before my run.

Her reasoning for this was to help train my gut to tolerate food and prime myself for the workout.

I hesitated. She continued, "What are you struggling with?"

"I don't want to get fat." I was so sick of that belief. I can't believe that I just blurted it out.

Marni's wisdom prevailed, "Julie, let's focus less on your weight and more on your body—is your body working for you or against you?"

"Yes, I want to do that. How do I do that?" I wanted to let go of the belief that I needed to be a certain weight to run fast or to run better.

Marni continued, "I want you to focus on how you are feeling and assess what your body can do instead of what it looks like. This will allow you to better understand if you have limiters beyond weight."

I loved that she was focused on me as a person instead of my body mass index or my weight on the scale. She wanted me to keep these questions in mind as we worked together. "Do you have good energy for your workouts?" "Do you feel strong, resilient, and healthy?" "Are you able to recover well after your workouts?" "Are you feeling stronger, faster, or fitter?"

I loved these questions and was so grateful to be working with Marni. Not only was she extremely knowledgeable and passionate but she was also real and caring. Marni encouraged me to stop worrying about gaining weight and instead get to know my body. She was right. I would get so mad at my body. (*Reflecting on this now, I see how this was one of the contributors to my pain.*)

I was gaining confidence every day planning my daily diet and balancing each meal. It was getting easier. I sent my sheets to Marni so she could take a peek to ensure I was on track. I liked this accountability as well. I needed it. I didn't want to fall back into my old habits and it was nice to have her support and encouragement when I felt that pushback.

Marni noticed that I left the pre- and post-workout sections empty on the sheet. I confessed that I wasn't eating anything before my runs or after.

She encouraged me to start, "This will help you get the most out of your body for each workout."

I wasn't sure what to eat before a run and she suggested applesauce or a few saltine crackers. I later found a banana also worked as an option.

Taking in nutrition 30 minutes before a run wasn't easy to adopt. My habit had been to get up early, sneakers laced, and out the door. Food was not on my mind and it was refreshing. It was the one moment I didn't think about food, yet Marni was coaching me to eat something before a run and to think about it. *Sigh.* It was not easy.

Many mornings, I would forget or I wouldn't allow enough time. Given I was only running five miles some mornings, I told myself that I didn't need to eat anything. Yet the more I worked with Marni the more aware I became of the sentences that were contributing to my poor relationship with food — sentences I needed to question and confront. My belief system was holding me back not only with my relationship with food but my relationship with myself. This was the biggest change I wanted to make. The relationship I had with myself. It was not kind or loving. It was critical and mean.

As a mother, I didn't want this part of me to be passed down to my children. I wanted to teach them how to have healthy, loving relationships and that meant I needed to start with myself— I had work to do.

***

My children loved the applesauce pouches and I found those to be perfect to place next to my clothes as a reminder to eat before I ran. I had to try something and laying things out the night before was already an established habit for me—why not add the food too?

Every night before I went to bed I placed my running clothes out in the bathroom along with an applesauce pouch or a banana. I would eat before I got my clothes on to run. It was a change. I would need to get up a little earlier to make sure I ate something but I told Marni I would and my determination and integrity overpowered my fear.

I was happy to tell her I was starting to feel better. I was improving the planning of my meals and was surprised how fast I took this on. Her coaching and food ideas empowered me and I felt more energetic. I was cooking and baking and my children were watching and helping. I forgot how much I loved to do both. I was turning a corner. I was on my way to building a better relationship with food and my body.

The next time Marni and I talked, she asked how I was feeling. I told her I was eating a bit before my runs and my stomach was tolerating it well. However, I was having a hard time with my longer runs. I was experiencing a lot of gastrointestinal distress mid-way through my runs. When I mentioned this, she asked about what I was using for hydration and nutrition during my long runs. She suspected it may be the products I was using that were causing a problem. She recommended a hydration product for me to try and believed that would be better for my sensitive stomach. This particular product was for both hydration and fueling.

I made the switch. I would fill my bottles up and place them in my hydration vest for my long runs. I stopped using gels to see how my body responded to the hydration alone. I loved the taste and for the next several long runs I felt great. I had no urge to use the bathroom, and no stomach cramping or discomfort. I was thrilled.

Chapter Six
Default Stories

Aware of the voice living
inside my head. She isn't kind
or encouraging—
rather judgy, full of fear.
I tell her to sit down,
put up her feet,
here— *have some tea*—
while I decide
what else is available to me?

The power of curiosity
comes through.
What else could be true?
Questioning my brain's
default story—a superpower
that's mine every time.
To make a shift—
interrupt the replay from
day to day.
An internal victory—
I say.

Sundays became the day I planned and prepared meals. I opened the meal-planning document Marni had sent me. My stomach was in knots.

This isn't a test Julie.

I would get so nervous as I filled in breakfast, lunch, and dinner including snacks and pre-and post-workout foods.

I hope I'm doing this right. I hope I'm adding in enough food. Why is this so hard?

I would type then delete and then type, then second guess myself, and delete again.

It would take me over an hour to plan my meals. I was learning and unlearning what I'd thought about food most of my life—not as a way to nourish me and keep me healthy but as something I needed to earn. When I got stuck, I would look at the documents she provided me with food options…add rice, noodles, and sweet potato. Carbohydrates and healthy fats were essential. Her voice would creep in and reassure me as I wrote down my meals.

I would check that each meal was balanced with carbohydrates, protein, and fat. I was completing the pre- and post-workout sections as well. I wrote that I would have applesauce or a banana with water before I ran, and a handful of raw nuts and banana with some drink within 30 minutes post-workout.

I would then send it off to Marni so she would get another snapshot of my week and see how I was doing. Ultimately, the goal was to get to a point when I felt confident enough to do this on my own. It needed to become a habit, a lifestyle with less time and effort to plan my meals. I was hoping I would get to this point. Yet, in the first month of working with Marni, I had my doubts. It was hard because my brain was battling with old stories and beliefs about food. I wanted to believe in this new story but it was challenging.

How did I get to this point? How did I let myself buy into all the nonsense that carbohydrates were bad?

I wanted to be healthy, strong, and resilient. I wanted to be running until my last breath. Yet, this belief that carbohydrates would make me fat was not going to work. If I wanted to be a healthy, strong, resilient runner for life, I would need to let go of that idea.

My therapist whom I was seeing in addition to Marni challenged me on this thinking. I was working with her at the same time. I needed the space to process what Marni was coaching me on and the cognitive dissonance I was experiencing. The thought that carbohydrates would make me fat was a belief I wanted and needed to let go of. It was my brain's default story. I was glad to be aware of this—because I could decide if I wanted to keep believing this or not. I began to question this story—*What else could be true?*

Marni was providing me with the information, support, and knowledge to answer this question. It was a way for me to shift my mindset. My body needed carbohydrates. This macronutrient provides the best source of energy—fueling my brain and central nervous system, helping my mood and sleep, and improving my digestive system—just to list a few truths.

What else could be true?

Carbohydrates were important to add to my daily diet because they would fuel me in my racing, would delay fatigue, and assist with fat metabolism.

In Marni Sumbal's book, *Essential Sports Nutrition: A Guide to Optimal Performance for Every Active Person,* she writes "Adequate carbohydrate intake can safeguard your glycogen storage and protein stores and support blood sugar levels during exercise, helping you sustain energy during your hard workouts and protect your immune system. The research on carbohydrates may look conflicting but if you prioritize real, wholesome, nutrient-dense sources of food instead of processed, refined, nutrient-poor sources, you, too, can experience great performance without sabotaging your health or body composition goals."

The more I read her book, the more excited and eager I became to adopt this lifestyle.

***

Marni's coaching made an immediate impact on my life. Not only was I understanding another contributor to my gastrointestinal symptoms and stomach pain but I was also acknowledging my default stories around food, body image, and being a mother runner by asking myself better questions. It was powerful. Rather than beating myself up over and over which was my default action, I questioned and prayed. Questioning allowed a shift each day for me to decide if the story was worth repeating and meditating on God's word allowed me to understand Him, His truth, and how He wanted me to respond.

My brain could be so confident and so matter-of-fact, yet so much of my thinking was outdated and no longer serving me. I was noticing how my increased awareness about my relationship with food was shifting by the power of curiosity. Questioning these old thought loops was a way to confront these old stories. This tool of awareness and questioning was not only beneficial for me in facing my relationship with food but also for everything in my life — including running. When negative thoughts took over — *You don't belong here, You're not fast enough or good enough.* — it allowed me to ask, *What else could be true? What does God say I am?* I didn't want to be neglectful of God. I needed to turn to the Lord for help and to seek Him. This wasn't something I could do myself.

They say the mind is our most powerful tool. I could attest to this.

What was I going to choose to take root in my mind?

I was praying for the Lord's guidance, to turn away from my sinful behavior and thoughts. During my healing, I was starting to reap the rewards. My body was feeling stronger on my runs and I noticed more energy throughout the day. I was also recovering faster after my long runs compared to before. I was on my way to building a healthy relationship with food and with myself.

Managing my mind and meal planning went hand in hand. Each Sunday, when I would sit down to plan my meals for the week, I noticed the thoughts. Aunt Phoebe with her squeaking voice and fear tactics would show up.

That's too many carbs. How many calories is that? That's too much food to be eating.

The old thought patterns would float to the surface. This time instead of shoving them back down or agreeing, I nodded and took a deep breath.

I can do this. Yes, we used to think that carbohydrates were not good but now we think differently.

Carbohydrates would be my best energy source for running and I would eat balanced meals to be healthy, happy, and strong.

I went back to my *why*—my children and my future self. I would not pass down my default stories about food to my son or daughter. I would not sabotage my happiness or health by counting calories or tracking my weight anymore. I was in a position to teach my children—to help them establish a healthy relationship with food and I took this role very seriously.

I had the knowledge to take into the kitchen to prepare healthy balanced meals for myself and my family and the confidence to teach my children to not be misled by diet trends, fads, and the diet industry.

I was starting to write a new story for myself.

I am becoming the person who believes healthy food is my fuel for my workouts and to assist in my recovery after long hard runs. I'm committed to preparing healthy meals daily to be happy, healthy, and strong. I will treat my relationship with food as I do my relationship with myself and my family.

I was missing this piece for many years. I'm forever grateful for Marni guiding me and that our paths crossed.

When Marni and I ended our time together, I felt tremendous gratitude and appreciation for her guidance and support. I knew deep down I was going to be okay. I had the foundation of my daily diet dialed in and my mindset was in a healthier place. I would lean on this new knowledge Marni provided me as I moved forward. During times of challenge or when my inner judge, Aunt Phoebe, would squeak in with her protective ways, I would pay attention. I would not forget what I learned and I would look back at my progress with Marni. I had an awareness that I didn't have before. I was learning to question my thinking and had the tools and strategies to help me with a great team in my corner—Marni, Joel, my therapist, and the greatest member of all—God.

As I reflect, I find it interesting that I believed not eating or restricting my calorie intake would help me run stronger and faster. I had no fuel or not enough—yet I believed by getting the scale to that magic number I would be a better runner. Where did I get these beliefs from? I had my ideas. It makes me sad when I still hear, "You need to lose 10 or 15 pounds and you will be better at your sport." I'm grateful to Marni for teaching me to look at myself as a person instead of allowing the scale to determine my worth. Her philosophy was never about weight or a number—it was about how does your body feel? It was working with her that I realized food wasn't the problem, it was my thinking and beliefs about food.

Chapter Seven
Racing Back On

BIB number in place

13.1-mile race

Toe the start line

Pack it in.

Ready—

Go!

Big grin.

Weave in and out

Fall into pace

Breathe. Relax. Run

Breathe. Relax. Run

A mantra to say

Look!

All the runners are here to play.

Cheers and shouts charge the air

Goosebumps in awe,

Body and mind aware

Energy rush for the miles ahead

Delight in the glow

Comeback power

You got this, Yo!

Races began to open back up on the calendar at the beginning of 2021. Vaccines were available to everyone in the United States and it was a great sign. My faith that Boston would happen also grew. I couldn't wait to run the course that so many women I had admired ran. Women whose courage, persistence, and strength allowed this dream for me.

I got goosebumps as I imagined running the streets that Kathrine Switzer, Bobbi Gibb, Joan Benoit Samuelson, and Lynn Jennings ran. These women covered the walls of my bedroom as a child. These were the women I wanted to be. It was going to happen in 2021. I would get my chance to run from Hopkinton to Boston.

Coach Joel and I began making a plan for races to enter before October. It was important to work on speed and get back into racing mode. Last year was interesting for me as all races were switched to a virtual option, meaning you ran at any location, outside or on a treadmill, alone or with a group of friends. You ran based on an honor system. It was nice that you still got the medal and shirt but it wasn't the same. I truly missed the atmosphere of racing. All runners piled together, elbow to elbow at the start line, music filling our ears, the spectators, volunteers, police officers, and chip timing were things I took for granted—2020 gave me a new perspective on racing.

Race directors were getting the green light to offer in-person racing however new rules and modifications were implemented. Races were opting for fewer participants, arrival times were based on a staggered start, and masks were mandatory before the start of the race and at the start line. During racing registration, a new option was required to be completed. There were 15-minute increments from which to choose so that runners would be staggered, no longer all starting together in a crowd. Social distancing was still recommended.

I didn't think these new rules for racing would impact me much at all. Yet when the first half marathon I signed up for at the end of March was a go, my mind was preoccupied with the new rules. Fear stepped in.

With all these new rules, are you sure you want to race right now? This is crazy. Do you think this is worth it?

My thoughts began to spiral.

Okay, so when can I get there? Will I be able to take the mask off when I run? Will my family be able to come to cheer me on?

I had a lot of questions. I felt the tension in my body—my stomach tightening, my breath turned shallow—panic and anxiety were front and center. More questions filled my head. The constant worry about other runners and what they were doing or thinking was consuming me. It made me not want to race.

I'm okay with standing next to people but are they? Do I want to do this? Do I want to show up?

These questions were taking up a lot of brain energy and I felt it in my body.

I was glad I recognized these thoughts and feelings and reached out to my coach. I was glad when Joel mentioned this new dynamic of racing, that as a runner we are now thinking about this other element that we never had to think about and it was okay to think about these things. I was relieved he said that. *Coach, can you read my mind?*

I felt lighter after we talked. The elephant in the room was confronted and I didn't need to explain myself. He knew. He understood. I was grateful. Once again, I was thankful to have him in my corner. His validation and reassurance were helpful and a great reminder that what I was feeling and thinking wasn't crazy. I was human.

***

I was getting excited to toe the start line for the next race on the calendar, The Mad Cow 5k in Nelson, NY. This was my first 5K race since April 2019. The best part was that my son, Brindsley, was going to run it too. I told him I wouldn't be running with him but just ahead of him. He was excited to run by himself and had no problem with me running without him. Racing rules were changing week by week, and I was glad to hear that we would all be starting at the same time.

The race course was over country roads, and rolling hills, with open fields for miles. There was a chance of a mad cow chasing you.

I'm in! I'm joking about the mad cow but the name got me to sign up.

Felicia, Brindsley, and I placed ourselves at the front of the pack for the start.

Why not? I'm racing this one, don't hold back.

It was awesome to have everyone together again on the start line. Runners of all ages lined up for the start at 9 a.m. I was happy to see so many kids Brindsley's age there. The temperature was climbing and it was already 80 degrees. I looked over at Brindsley, his blue eyes were soaking it all in.

He looked up at me with a big smile on his face, "Mom, this is going to be fun."

I smiled, "Yes, Brindsley, this is going to be so much fun, and look at all the kids you get to run with."

I was happy to be sharing the love of running with Brindsley. Jeff, Delaney, and my mom were there to cheer us on. They were along the side of the road to see us start. The announcer shouted, "I will count down from three then you will hear the blowhorn." Three, two, one… honk! We were off. I got nudged in the arm by a fellow runner and it made me grateful to be racing again with fellow runners. Felicia and I were in the lead pack with four other women.

Wow, this is awesome to have so many of us together up front. Julie, relax and stick with the group.

My mind started to chatter.

It's *so hot, and this pace is fast.*

I took charge.

I'm racing. Push yourself. It's supposed to be fast. It's only three miles then you're done. You got this.

I shook out my arms and kept my eyes on the woman ahead of me. They pulled ahead but I stayed calm. I had two more miles to go.

Get up these hills. Pump your arms. A downhill is up next.

I kept coaching myself. I made it up the last hill, took a sharp left turn, and went downhill. Just what I needed. I used gravity to my advantage, leaned forward, and flew down letting my legs carry me. The finish line was just around the corner.

I heard cheers from voices I recognized. I glanced over to the left and saw Jeff, Delaney, and my mom shouting "Go, Julie, you got this!"

Perfect timing, I needed a pick-me-up. Their cheers and shouts gave me a surge of energy as I picked up my pace around the corner. I heard cowbells ringing—*I need more cowbell*—my mind flashed to Saturday Night Live and Will Ferrell. I giggled to myself as I passed a large crowd of people cheering.

There was the finish line. Thank goodness. I kicked it in with all I had left.

I hunched over, my hands collapsed to my knees, and sweat dripped from my hat. I closed my eyes.

Thank you body, thank you mind for another race, another finish.

I grabbed some water and met up with Felicia. We went to cheer on Brindsley.

I looked past the finish and around the corner was Brindsley. I was so surprised to see him already. "WOW! Go Brindsley Go! Kick it in. Give it all you got." His face was full of determination, his arms pumped and his legs dashed to the finish.

Look at him go!

Felicia and I ran over to meet him. I was so proud of how well he ran. I wrapped my arms around him in a big sweaty hug. We did it! "Mom, I beat my time from the last race" with an enormous smile, he hugged me again. "Brindsley, yes, you did and you are amazing no matter your time. Did you have fun?"

"Yes mom I did, I even walked a little" he smirked.

"I'm so glad you had fun. I did too." I squeezed his hand. "Let's go find Dad, Delaney, and Nana."

***

It was September 4, 2021. The Gorges Ithaca Half Marathon race was today. This was my last race leading up to The Boston Marathon. The course was flat and fast. The weather looked perfect as I grabbed my bag to head out. The night before I packed my gear—a hydration vest, two soft flasks, three energy gels, a change of clothes, extra sneakers, socks, a water bottle, and a hydration mix. I didn't like to rush on race day so I was happy. I had my bag all ready to go.

I was excited to see where I was at in my training and looked forward to racing. The race was a staggered start with runners grouped at designated times—we signed up for the time slot when we registered for the race. This allowed a few runners to start together with others spaced out behind so there wasn't a crowd. We were back to social distancing without a formal start.

Felicia and I arrived early to pick up our bib numbers and warm up. We still had an hour before we would start the race according to the time slot we chose. As we made our way over to the tables, a group of runners was already heading out on the course. I was anxious to start the race as I watched them take off. I looked at Felicia, "Do you think we'll get in trouble if we start at a time slot we didn't register for?" She looked at me and grinned, "I was wondering the same thing." I laughed. Here we were grown women wondering if we would get in trouble for starting earlier than we signed up for. We started jogging around the starting area waiting for the announcer to call the next group of runners to begin. I was ready and didn't want to wait another 45 minutes to start. I could tell Felicia was feeling the same way. I recalled Bobbi Gibb and Kathrine Switzer—this was nothing compared to the ruckus they made, "Let's go for it!" I looked at Felicia and she agreed. *Heck, when did I ever break the rules?* "We are such rebels", we laughed and kept our ears alert for the next time slot to begin.

We heard the announcer and headed over to the start line. I would admit it was awkward not having a large group of people to start with but I was getting used to it. I was glad Felicia was with me.

"Ready to go?" I turned to Felicia as we got closer to the start line.

She nodded.

Our feet crossed over the start, and we heard the small beep of our chip timer—the race was on. We were on the clock. I normally started my watch when I began a race yet today I forgot it. No matter— today's race goal was not about time but nutrition timing. I loved that I didn't beat myself up about my watch—a huge win for me.

My first goal was to focus on my nutrition timing. *Take in sips of hydration every mile one gel at mile five, and the other gel at mile ten.* My focus was to nail down my nutrition for this half marathon to prepare me for Boston. My second goal for the race was to run the second half faster than the first.

During the first mile, I swallowed a bug—yuck. This was the third bug in the last month that had decided to fly into my mouth—*I'm not joking. It's making me wonder.* Anyway, it was stuck in my throat for a bit, leading to a coughing attack—not how I imagined starting a race. I wore my running vest with fluids and could flush it down my throat as I continued to run. I laughed it off instead of getting irritated. I guess I needed a little extra protein to start the race.

I kept my eyes on the runners ahead of me and stayed calm as I turned the corner. To my right was a gorgeous view of the water and my body relaxed. Breathe, relax, run was my mantra as I acknowledged the scenery around me. I got to mile five taking in a gel and hydration keeping my focus on nutrition while staying relaxed. Around mile eight, a few runners passed me and my chest began to tighten. My arms felt heavy and my shoulders tensed. I felt rigid as I watched them pull ahead of me. I noticed it right away, the old Julie decided to show up and run with me.

Oh no, you are going too slow, you aren't good enough.

I knew what to do. I'd been practicing this in my training and visualization. This was an old narrative of mine, the fear of not performing as expected or anticipated. In the past, the mental aspect would affect my performance and I didn't know how to handle it. I've carried this around since high school cross country. Yet, over the years, I've done the work to confront this fear and manage my mind.

I was surprised it came up but I welcomed it. It was my chance to prove to myself that I could work through this. I shook my arms down by my side and took some deep breaths

Breathe, relax, run. Breathe, relax, run. There is nothing that's gone wrong here.

Then to my surprise I heard, *Julie, you are right where you need to be, you are a strong runner, and you have a strong mind.* What a gentle and kind thought. My body listened and the tension released.

In the last half of the race, I continued to coach myself with the mantras I'd practiced and kept my focus on nutrition timing. I was taking in hydration every mile and feeling strong. The temperature was rising as the sun beat down on my face, yet I didn't feel overheated or thirsty —I was right on point. Without my watch on I had no idea how fast or slow I was running —yet I wasn't worried. For the last three miles of the race, I kept my eyes ahead of the runners in front of me. I challenged myself to see how many runners I could catch until the finish. *Let's see what I can do,* as I picked up my pace. Cheers and shouts got louder as I turned the corner. I heard a spectator shout, "The finish is up ahead, you are almost there!"

I saw the finish line. *Let's go!* I pumped my arms and picked up my pace to finish strong—*give it all you got.* I had no idea what time I came in yet when I finished I was happy. I managed my mind, nailed my nutrition plan, and felt confident going into Boston next month. I went into this race with two goals— to focus on nutrition timing and to run the second half of the race faster than the first half. I was able to execute my plan and the result was a personal record—36 days until The Boston Marathon!

***

I was tired when I got home. I didn't want to do anything but lie down and put my feet up.

Oh wait, I'm a mother of two very active children so this was very unlikely.

"Hey, mom, will you come out and play football with me?"

I groaned inside as I just stepped into the house. I wanted to put my feet up, close my eyes, and reflect on the race.

"Yes, Brindsley, of course. Let me change my sneakers and I will be right out."

I made a promise to myself early on in parenting that running or racing wouldn't be an excuse to not show up for my children. My family would be my priority so when I chose to go out for long runs or enter a race I made sure I was ready for my children when I got back. I was not sure how much longer play time with mom would be cool or fun so I pushed the groan aside. I let gratitude fill me up.

They are growing up so fast. My son wants me to play with him and I'm healthy and strong to do so.

I headed outside. He told me the teams and instructed me on the play we would run. He hiked me the ball. I found the energy to run and play. What a great way to work out my soreness. I found the more I played with Brindsley, laughed, and smiled, the better my legs felt and my heart was full.

***

As I reflected on the Gorges Half Marathon, I was proud I was able to put my mental training into action. I was prepared leading up to the race physically. It was my mind that was the player to manage—*negative thoughts swirl in and out and if I'm not aware those thoughts can spiral out of control.* When a few runners passed me early on, I panicked. I felt my shoulders rise, and my chest and back tighten. I was happy to notice. I began talking to myself calmly and encouragingly. *It's okay they passed me. Breathe, relax, and run my race.* I was surprised my body responded the way it did yet I know why. My fear of not doing well, of coming in last, of not meeting expectations. I was so proud of not beating myself up and staying calm. I was talking like a supportive coach the entire race. *I got this, you're right on pace, keep looking ahead and see how many runners you can catch.* I wasn't freaking out and if I started to I was able to redirect my self-talk to the mantras I'd been practicing. *YES!* This was a great brain triumph for me. The practice and the hard work were paying off.

I didn't go into this race feeling tremendous pressure about my time. My main goal and focus were on nutrition. I was able to accomplish this and my brain stayed focused on the task. This was good for me to recognize, I can have other goals in a race other than time or pace. It did help that I forgot my watch. It wasn't beeping at me and I wasn't looking at it. *I wonder if I will wear my watch in Boston.*

A week later I received an email from the Boston Athletic Association. Every time I saw their name in my email I felt a mix of emotions. *Please don't tell me the race is canceled. Please be an email confirming the weekend events.* I stared at my inbox, moved the cursor over the subject title, and clicked. I scanned the email for words I feared — *cancel, a virtual option only or we regret to inform you* —none. I went back to the top of the email to read it with a smile on my face.

A Boston Marathon app would be available for friends and family to track me on October 11, 2021 — race day. The email was explaining how to share, download, and use the app. I was so excited to send this email to my coach, family, and friends. My confidence soared — The Boston Marathon was a go and any further communication from the Boston Athletic Association would be to get us ready for race day.

Chapter Eight
Mantra Runner

Darkness thick.
The right foot follows out
into the warm morning.
Make a run for it
I say
Before my mind
gets in the way.
I can't wait for her—
don't give her time
to catch up.
Her squeaky voice
interrupts—
Stay in bed,
It's too dark out
Run another time.
We've had a good run
Yet—I've retrained my mind.
Run first, don't think
Clothes laid out
Sneakers at the door
Run loop ready
Slip out—

Make a run for it!
my body shouts.
Clouds hide the stars
Where is the moon?
I look up into the darkness
There she is
Good morning Moon.
Let's make a run for it!
It will be light soon.

I hopped out of bed at 4:30 a.m. A 45-minute run was planned with 25 minutes of strength training after. Boston was getting closer and my excitement was growing as I counted down the weeks. I grabbed my reflective gear and headed out the door. It was dark and cloudy, with no stars to shine my way. The warm breeze hit my face and the quietness was soothing. The road was without any street lights, just my light to guide me.

As I got closer to the village, the street lights illuminated my way and my eyes adjusted to the brightness. It allowed me to look up more frequently instead of staring at the ground. All I heard were birds as I looked around and noticed my surroundings. No cars, no trucks, only stillness, and peace. I loved this about running in the early mornings. The sound of my breath and my feet hitting the pavement. A time to check in with my thoughts and clear my mind. It was a space to practice not only running but my mindset.

My journey to get here has taught me to be aware of my thoughts. There was a time I was burdened with a false sense of who I was which led to many years of pain. It was my responsibility to check in and pay attention to my thoughts each day. What would I think about? What thoughts would I cultivate? Someone once told me that our minds were like a garden. What did I want to plant and grow in my mind? I was the gardener and it was my job to be aware of what I was focusing on. What would I read, listen to, and watch, and how would I talk to myself? What words would I meditate on each day? Were they helpful, kind, true, or something I would say to a friend? I needed to be deliberate about what I would think about each day. I wanted to remove the noxious weeds from my mind. A scripture verse that helped me was Romans 12:2 which reads, "Do not conform to the pattern of this world but be transformed by the renewing of your mind. Then you will be able to test and approve what God's will is—his good, pleasing and perfect will." This was what I wanted to take root in my garden. I could take control over what I thought about with God's guidance. I saw how much it mattered. My children were watching me. Listening to me. *What would I say to them?*

I would say—*You are robust, adaptable, and strong.*

I would say—*You are unique and valuable.*

I would say—*You are made for this.*

It's going to take practice, patience, and courage. Will it be easy? NO. Yet God is with you and His spirit lives inside of you. GO. GO. GO.

***

Marathon training and racing had taught me a lot about the importance of a mantra.

When I'm tired, what will I say to myself to keep going?

My brain said, "I needed to stop."

When I feel the pain, the nerve twinges, what would I say?

My brain yelled, "I needed to slow down."

When I let my brain spiral to negative thinking without fighting back, my performance suffered. I needed a mantra to stop the spiral. I was practicing what I would say when I raced The Boston Marathon. I had a list of thoughts I repeated to myself to keep my brain calm and my body relaxed. I'd accepted that running a marathon would be painful. I would hurt. I would get tired. My brain would tell me to slow down and would ask me why I was running. I'd been here before and I knew that pain didn't always mean harm.

This was part of the racing experience I'd come to know and love. It made me stay curious about what my body could do.

I hurt but if I just keep going what is possible? If I can manage my mind, hold on just a bit longer, get to the edge, and respect it, what will I learn about myself?

Running has allowed me to answer these questions. I was capable of more than I realized and racing gave me evidence of that.

We may not have a great race every time we toe the line yet in each race we learn something new about ourselves. Something that we can reflect on for the next run and something we can improve on. This is life. When things don't go as planned what will the gift or silver lining be? Trust me, there will be one, look hard to find it.

***

I remember one Monday morning my alarm went off at 5 a.m. *Time to run.* I lay in bed listening to the rain outside. My mind began to chatter.

It's raining out. Stay in bed. You can run later.

I knew better. Those thoughts were strong and loved to creep in. This time I just laughed. I would get up and run no matter the weather. This was my time and I felt so much better when I finished a run.

I jumped out of bed and started getting ready. I continued to coach myself.

I love running in the rain and Boston is just a few weeks away. Who knows what the weather will bring? This is great training.

I stepped outside and a fresh earthy smell filled my nostrils. I took a deep breath in. I loved that smell. All the creeks roared as I passed them on the road. I had a negative split 50-minute run—25 minutes out, 1-minute walk, and then 25 minutes back at a faster pace. It was dark and cloudy, just my light shining the way as water splashed up with each stride. Boston was less than eight weeks away. The thought gave me the chills and a burst of energy overtook my legs as I picked up the pace. It was time to get moving, 25 minutes back. This was the training that mattered. I believed this more and more and it brought joy and fun back to my running.

Chapter Nine
My Brain While Running

Eyes down lost in thought
A to-do list runs through my mind
with each stride. Nature neglected.
My sneakers scuff the ground—
A rock trips me up, *pay attention.*

Sunshine peeks between the bare
limbs of maple and hickory.
My posture shifts— head up,
eyes alert. The warm glow relaxes
my face, and my jaw unclenches.

I shake my arms out and breathe.
The glorious sun wakes me up—
nudges me out of my self-absorption.
Mindfulness returns. Squirrel chatters,
and blue jay whistles as I run past.

The sun was just coming up when I headed out the lobby
doors. The warm air hit my face as I took in my new surroundings. *Which way do I go?* I looked up the road with lots
of traffic and no shoulder for me to run on. I looked down

to see more space with lots of side streets, shops, and exploring, *down it is.* I pressed the start button on my watch and off I went. *I'll head out for 30 minutes then turn around and come back. That will work for today.*

My family and I were in Asheville, North Carolina visiting my sister. Our first trip out of New York since 2019 and it felt great to be in a new place. I was excited to explore new roads and take in the sights. This was the benefit of running, you could head outdoors anywhere at any time. I didn't have any excuse not to train. My coach sent my training plan for the week and I knew exactly what to do. The hotel had a large open weight room. This made it easy for me on the days I had strength training or yoga. I would follow the schedule then the rest of the day would be with my family. I was happy to get up early and get going. It was how I was made.

Yet my brain likes to butt in, *you're on vacation, you don't have to run. Taking a few days off won't hurt your training, you already made it to Boston.*

Where would I be with those thoughts—not crossing the finish at The Boston Marathon. I rolled my eyes at those sentences. I countered back, *I am on vacation and I get to run. I'm training for The Boston Marathon and I will follow the training plan my coach sent. I made it to Boston and I will prepare my body for the challenging course.* I smiled as I leaned forward, pumped my arms, and climbed the next hill. *I'm training for the Boston Marathon.*

I was happy to shift my mindset. I was proud of myself. I recognized the sentences that could send me in a spiral. I was deliberate with my self-talk and thrilled to see my hard work paying off once again.

***

I recalled one Saturday morning training run. It was 13 miles with one-mile repeats in the middle of the run. I made sure to wear my hydration vest to sip from my flask every 15 minutes. I carried one energy gel which I would consume at mile six. I was happy the gels I'd been racing and training with were agreeing with my stomach. I wasn't having any issues. This was a huge win and Marni was to thank.

I pushed the mile repeats hard and within the last 35 minutes, my body was talking to me. It showed up in my right hip, the hip that over the years has been out of sync. The discomfort got louder and traveled down to my knee. *Ugh.* I knew this pain yet I was annoyed it had shown up. I was hoping the gluten-free diet that I'd been on for almost a year now would immune me to feeling this. I felt myself getting irritated. I noticed and switched my thoughts.

Get back to the present.

I didn't want to go down the rabbit hole of beating myself up, an old habit of mine. My body was talking to me because I was running hard.

This pain is okay Julie, you know this pain. It's not harmful.

I stayed calm.

Okay, this is the perfect time to practice the thoughts I will need on race day. This is it. This pain may show up and I need to accept and decide what I'm going to do—let my thoughts get the best of me, tense up and freak out, or remember what I know about my body and mind and fight back. What would I say to myself to move through the pain and discomfort? What would I say to keep pressing on?

I took some deep breaths, looked ahead on the trail, and brought my attention to the trees, the breeze, and then my arms.

Shake out your arms. Relax your shoulders. Breathe, relax, and run, Julie. I have what it takes. I am a strong runner and I'm almost done. Keep going. This pain doesn't mean stop.

The more I ran and coached myself, the pain stayed the same, it didn't get worse and it didn't get better yet I was able to keep pace with Felicia. I was able to keep running without changing my form and keep a good attitude.

The discomfort stayed the same and was acceptable to me. I relaxed knowing I wasn't harming myself and my running form had not changed... *YES!* I was so proud of myself because not that long ago when this same discomfort came on, my performance went sideways. It was when I ran the virtual Boston Marathon in 2020. I didn't manage my mind. I had a hard time redirecting my thoughts and my attitude.

The pain took over and I gave into my self-doubt, worry, and fear,— my inner judge controlled the race.

Not this time, I was armed with the truth. This pain didn't mean slow down, or harm, I could keep going. I focused on my nutrition intake and mantras. I'd been practicing for this very moment. I was glad it was happening so I had the evidence that I could keep going.

Hey, we are safe. We are running. This is what we love to do. I'm going to stay calm and keep my brain in the game. The discomfort didn't get worse and this was my green light—*Keep going. Keep pushing.* We got to the end of the trail and finished the 13-mile run. This was a victory!

We finished with a five-minute cool-down walk and wouldn't you know, all the discomfort was gone. The nerve pain stopped. My right hip felt almost like my left hip and my right knee was completely fine. So weird, yet so amazing! This was the evidence I needed. I could handle this discomfort. The confidence in myself and my body was improving. I was capable of so much. I went into the run with proper fueling and a good attitude. I was able to manage my mind. I was learning that my body will do what my mind asked of it when taken care of.

I believe this not only helps with running but with life. Are you curious about what you say to yourself during troubles or challenges—it matters. Pay attention when you're out on the road. I find it's the best place to escape the noise of the world, unplug, and get to know your thoughts. Don't be afraid to question what comes up. What else could be true? Or if you're a Christian like me, what does God say I am?

Chapter Ten
Pivot and Adapt

Boston Marathon is two weeks away
and a cold has found its way.
My throat is sore,
I got the sniffles—
even my right leg has the niggles.
I won't fret
or get upset.
I will be kind to my body and mind
As my immune system fights back
I'll do my best to keep my training on track
I will prioritize rest
Eat nutritious foods
Keep an optimistic mood
I won't let this get me down
This is temporary
And I'll come around

The Hughes home was down and out. Noses were running and tissue boxes were flying. The children started back to school. Two weeks in and Delaney was home sick with a fever. She was not allowed back until she got a COVID test and was symptom-free for five days. I called around to find a place to get her tested while praying she was negative.

I learned that one of our local hospitals had a clinic set up just for testing. I took Delaney hoping we would find out the results soon—Boston was so close. *What if she's positive?* I didn't even want to think about it. We arrived at the clinic and it appeared that we weren't the only ones in need of the test. Several people were sitting outside the waiting room and standing along the hallway waiting to be called. We signed in and the gentleman told us to wait in the car until they called my phone to come back in. Delaney and I headed back to the parking garage to wait. She wasn't happy. She didn't feel well. I felt bad for rushing over here instead of letting her rest first but I thought it was the best thing to do.

"Mom, I want to go home. Is this going to hurt?" she asked looking very distressed.

"Delaney, I want to go home too but this is needed so you can get back to school. It will be a quick tickle up your nose with a swab and I'll be right next to you."

My phone rang. We had permission to check in by the clinic doors. I took Delaney's hand as we walked down the crowded hallways. There were so many people. I reached for my mask making sure it was snug on my face. I didn't want to get COVID. The nurse was kind and gentle and ushered us into the small cubicle. The swab was in and out of Delaney's nose before she had a moment to resist.

"That didn't hurt at all mom."

I took Delaney's hand and squeezed her, "You are so brave. You did great."

The nurse told us the results would be on the patient portal tomorrow. We hurried back to the car weaving through the line of people waiting for testing. I couldn't believe all the people in line. I turned to Delaney, "Let's go home and sleep." She nodded as we picked up our pace to the car.

My training continued. I prayed my immune system stayed strong as I cared for Delaney. I checked the patient portal that night even though the nurse told me the results wouldn't be in until tomorrow. *Sigh!* I was praying she was negative meanwhile, my body was starting to talk to me. My throat was scratching and my nose began to run.

Oh no, am I getting a cold?

The Boston Marathon was two weeks away and I was praying my body would fight off whatever was coming.

Is this the start of COVID? Oh boy, I hope not.

I checked the computer again to see if Delaney's results were in. No, the nurse said the results wouldn't be posted until the morning yet here I was checking every 10 minutes anyways. I laughed at my impatience. I would try to get some sleep and check the first thing before my run.

My alarm went off the next morning and the first thought that popped into my mind was about Delaney's COVID test results. I jumped out of bed and headed to the computer. I pleaded to God, as I was navigating the website and clicking to find the page.

Please have her test be negative. Please have her test be negative.

I scanned the screen to find the words negative next to her name.

Phew! Thank you, Lord. Delaney's COVID-19 test was negative. Her test results kept my spirits up and I was convinced that what I had was just a cold.

I prioritized sleep, hydration, and rest but continued my training the best I could. If I needed to back off a bit I would. My training had been solid up until now. A few days of adjusting the schedule would be okay and my coach agreed. It wouldn't set me back. My inner judge, good old Aunt Phoebe, thought the opposite.

You shouldn't be running at all. You probably have COVID. If you do have it, you might not be able to travel to Boston.

She was such a pain in the butt.

I didn't want to spiral, it would only make me feel worse — so I fought back.

Here Aunt Phoebe, have a cup of tea and put your feet up. This cold is temporary. I'll bounce back and be ready for Boston.

I was deliberate with my thoughts, working hard to turn them around and keep optimistic.

Two days later I was back at the clinic with Brindsley. He had a fever and was sent home from school. We both signed in to get tested. I didn't have a fever but I still felt off. I was confident we were both negative. We had to be.

If COVID is the reason we can't travel to Boston I will be furious.

We both got the swab up our noses then we were back in the car.

Brindsley laughed, "That tickled my nose mom."

I smiled, "Mine too, and made my eyes water. Let's pray we are negative okay."

"Okay mom, I will."

The next day Brindsley had no fever and was back to himself. Delaney had one more day of quarantine then she would return to school. My runs were the only thing that kept me sane during the week my children were sick. Having both of them home tested my patience. They were feeling well enough to fight and argue again. Luckily for me, my throat was still sore and yelling wasn't an option. God had such a great sense of humor. He knew I didn't like to yell— I appreciated this scratching throat.

I opened my computer and navigated the site to find out the results. I said a quick prayer before I clicked on the link. I got to Brindsley's results first.

Negative, yes!

I looked for my results.

Negative. Thanks be to God! Boston Marathon here we come.

Chapter Eleven
Heart of Gratitude

Pumpkin waffles three piled high
Celebrating another Saturday
long run. Thank you body.
Aunt Phoebe (*my inner judge*) is
sitting across the table.
Her squeaky voice interrupts
my celebration.
You're going to eat ALL three waffles —
Isn't that a little too much?

I politely nod and reply —
thank you for noticing but yes,
yes, three is the right amount
for me today. She crosses her arms
over her chest as I open the jar
of almond butter.
I pick up the knife spreading
the delicious nut butter over each
waffle. Smooth clumps sit in
the nooks of each one.
My humming was interrupted by —
Don't overdo it. Almond butter

isn't fat-free ya know.

Aunt Phoebe just can't keep her
mouth shut—she speaks with
such confidence, such authority.
I smile and take a sip of my *bold* coffee.
Her voice is no longer mine.
I slice bananas and berries for
added sweetness to my plate.
I feel strong, happy, and resilient
as Aunt Phoebe melts away.

I couldn't wait to get a cup of coffee and put my feet up. I unlaced my sneakers, sweat dripping from my face and ponytail. I pulled off my socks taking a peek at my toenails—they were holding up pretty well this time around. I'd only had one toenail come off since training started and only a few that were black. *Thank you body, we did a great job today.* I was happy and grateful for the miles—it has been such a long process to get here.

I just finished my last long run before Boston—18 miles with an elevation gain of 1300 feet. I was tired. I was glad to be done yet what a beautiful morning for a long run. The view was breathtaking. The fall colors energized me up the hills—*what will I see next over the crest?* I loved running in the fall. This thought carried me for a while then I started thinking about breakfast.

I don't know why but when I run there is always a point in the miles when my mind trails to food. Does this happen to you?

Today's run was homemade gluten-free pumpkin waffles, and bananas with almond butter—some of my favorites and the motivation I needed to make the climbs today.

I walked into the kitchen. The smell of coffee hit my nose and I smiled. I loved that Jeff already had the coffee made. *He loves me even though I left him with the kids for over two hours.* I grabbed my coffee mug—"Strong vibes, Calm mind" was printed on it. This mug was a birthday gift from my children and one of my favorites. I filled it to the top and took a sip looking for Brindsley and Delaney. They were sitting on the couch watching a TV show. I interrupted their space with sweaty kisses and a good morning hug. It was great to see them. "Ugh mama, you are so sweaty" as they tried to keep their eyes on the TV screen dodging my kisses. I got the hint and headed to the kitchen table to eat.

Jeff sat with me as we had breakfast together and had a moment to talk. I felt these moments were rare and maybe this once I could be at peace with the kids watching TV. After all, it gave Jeff and me time to catch up on the week and check in with each other. I blurted out, "We head to Boston in six days! Can you believe it!" My excitement wasn't as contagious as I would like it to be but Jeff smiled as he sipped his coffee. He knew this was a big deal for me even if he didn't show it. I took a bite of my waffle as I reflected on the long road to get here. It wasn't easy. Yet, I can't imagine it happening any other way—the patience, perseverance, discipline, and mindset to keep going—paid off.

He doesn't have to be excited, I am and that's what matters. This is my dream. I began making a list in my mind of all the things I needed to get done before we headed to Boston. I reminded myself that as long as I had my race day clothes, sneakers, and gear nothing else mattered. Brindsley and Delaney headed into the kitchen, "How was your run mama?" I loved that they asked me.

"Fantastic! I found a penny and I saw two woolly bears on the side of the road."

"That's great mama," as they rushed off to play.

I sat back in my chair and sipped more coffee. My legs were sore as I propped them up. I was glad I had no stairs to climb. Today's run was challenging and a good test for me. I ran hard with huge elevation gains without nerve or hip discomfort. I didn't take the turn I was planning and ended up running a lot more elevation than I expected. It was interesting what happened. Aunt Phoebe showed up, *This is not the right way. You are overdoing it. Are you sure you want to run up all these hills?*

She was just looking out for me but I didn't need to believe every thought. I took charge. I would be ready for Heartbreak Hill.

This was a great confidence booster for Boston, this was just what I needed. I focused and practiced my mindset for the rest of the run. The route I ended up on was hard and Boston would be too. Yet, it was the evidence I needed to prove to myself that I was ready not only physically but mentally for The Boston Marathon. I had a new mindset and my faith was stronger than before. I knew the Lord would be with me. He would give me the strength I needed to make the climbs and cross the finish line. I was thrilled. My main goal was to finish with gratitude. I reminded myself no matter the outcome, gratitude! I would keep a heart of gratitude.

Chapter Twelve
BOSTON—It's Real

Believe in yourself
It's that simple
It doesn't need to be complicated
Though the whispers linger
Those mumbles are musty
Stale and uninspired
An old story on the shelf
Time to let go—I say
Leave it there and let it collect dust
You get to write a new story, *you must*
Take the leap
Deep inside your ready
You know what you're meant to do
Go for it!
I'm cheering for you.
 —You can do it!

We arrived in Boston on Friday at 2 p.m. The city was wild
with excitement as the countdown to the marathon was displayed at the finish line on Boylston Street. People were taking pictures and the streets were crowded. We spotted our

hotel, 250 feet from the finish line. This was the reason I picked this one. My family would be able to view the marathon and see the finish without having to move through the crowds or travel. It would also give me a chance to see my family cheering for me before I crossed the finish line.

We checked into the hotel. The staff greeted us with eye smiles and enthusiasm even with their masks on.

One of the women asked me, "Are you here to run The Boston Marathon?"

"Yes, I am! My first time here, I can't wait," my smile was wide under my mask.

Brindsley and Delaney were standing next to me trying to see over the counter.

"We have a little something for your kids." The woman came over to us and handed Brindsley and Delaney a stuffed animal. My children were on cloud nine. They loved stuffed animals. They were all smiles as they looked at each other discussing what they would name their bear. What a nice surprise. We grabbed our luggage and stepped into the next available elevator. We made sure our masks were in place. There was a mandate to wear masks in Boston while indoors. I was glad I packed a few extra cloth masks for the kids.

As we settled into the hotel room, I checked the schedule for the day. My top priorities were to show my vaccination status so I could go to the Expo to pick up my race packet and bib number. I was thrilled to go to the Expo and check out all the vendors and apparel. I couldn't wait to buy a shirt with the Boston Marathon logo on it.

I made my way to the enormous white tents set up two blocks away from the hotel. There were tables set up inside with a person at each table. I would need to verify that I had been vaccinated. I showed her my card and she placed a bracelet on my wrist that I had to wear the entire weekend.

"Don't take this off until you are done with the race."

I nodded and made sure it was snug. The bracelet was required to pick up my race packet at the Expo and to toe the start line on Monday. I looked down at the blue bracelet— *I get to run Boston in three days.*

I met back up with my family and we walked to the Expo. It was a few blocks away and my kids were excited to get out and move around. They were already complaining that they were bored. I took a deep breath. *They can be bored.* I didn't need to make it personal. Once we got walking, their attitude changed. Their eyes widen at the tall buildings, honking horns, people weaving around them, and the smells of tomato sauce and grilled meats. This was their first time in a big city and they were in awe.

Once we made it inside, the building was rather quiet.

Are we in the right place?

I spotted a sign instructing us to take the escalator for packet pick-up and the expo. My family and I stepped onto the escalator and, as we got to the top, the silence was filled with a bustle. We stepped off to see gatherings of people on our left and right. A volunteer was standing at the door to the entrance to packet pick up and ushered me in.

Wow, how fancy.

My family waited to the side while I walked up to the booth.

"Hello, I'm so excited to be here."

The woman and I exchanged happy glances and she said, "We are too. Welcome back."

"This is my first time running Boston, I can't wait." I leaned in closer to see what her name was on her tag.

"Do you have your bracelet and driver's license for identification?"

I handed her my driver's license and lifted my left arm so she could see my blue bracelet with the words 125th Boston Marathon on it. She nodded and began filing through the bib numbers and pulled out mine—10895. Several volunteers were behind her handing out clear plastic bags filled with coupons, goodies, and safety pins to attach the bib number. She instructed me to use this clear plastic bag for bag drop-off on race day.

"Thank you so much, Betty." I smiled and turned to see my family. Their patience was a blessing.

"Okay kids, let's go check out the clothing and goodies." I hoped this would excite them though they didn't look convinced.

Delaney turned to me, "This is so boring mom. When can we go?"

"I know this is boring for you, but I'm so glad you are here to cheer me on. Hang in there, after the marathon we have a few fun things planned for you. Trust me."

"Okay, mama," she agreed in her best grumbling voice.

I took her hand and we walked to the next room. In front of us was an enormous blue wall with yellow writing on it. The yellow writing was of all the names participating in the marathon.

"Kids, I need your help, see if you can find my name." They got excited then and we all headed to the wall to look.

"Mom, there it is!" Brindsley pointed to the wall.

I looked close, Julie Hughes. *There I am. What a special feeling to see my name among the other 20,000 entrants.*

Jeff got out his phone and took some pictures of us. There was a crowd of people now as we checked out the clothing and apparel. I wanted to buy one of each item I saw, luckily my family was with me to keep me in check. Brindsley picked out Spike, a unicorn stuffed animal with a yellow shirt. Delaney turned down the opportunity, which shocked me. I got her a cowbell instead, "look Delaney you can ring this to cheer us all on." She seemed content.

We headed to the next room where vendors were set up. One vendor had markers and posters for family and friends to make cheer signs—brilliant! Delaney and Brindsley marched right up to the table, picked up the colored markers, and got to work. In their best cursive writing, they filled the white sign trying to hide from me what they wrote.

"Mama, don't look, we want it to be a surprise!"

My heart was full as I watched them giggle and smile. I was so grateful they were here celebrating this marathon experience with me. They finished the signs and handed them to Jeff. I would get to see them after the marathon as they instructed. I couldn't wait! Who doesn't like any kind of handwritten note or poster in this case? It was so fun and special!

***

Boston was in two days! I tiptoed to the bathroom in hopes I wouldn't wake my family. I had a short run planned and was excited to check out the city. As I got ready, my son Brindsley peeked in and asked if he could run with me.

"Of course!" I love it when he wants to join me.

We both walked down to the hotel lobby and headed out to the busy morning streets. The city lights shined bright with every stride. Brindsley was in awe of the large, tall buildings and the noise all around us. I was too. Back home the roads were so quiet and dark. It was fun to have people up and moving with us. I could feel the energy of the city and we started chatting about what we saw.

"Mama, look at this building! Look at those lights! Why do those windows have bars on them?"

He was full of questions, excitement, and curiosity as we jogged down the street toward the finish line setup. As we got closer, a countdown to the start of the marathon was glowing at us... *Two days until the start.* I smiled, my dream was coming true and my family was here to enjoy it with me. I felt light on my feet as we continued past a gentleman who made conversation with us as we waited to cross the street. He was planning to run the marathon next year and was currently training to be an American Ninja Warrior. I was glad we stopped to chat with him and my son replied, "He was nice."

"Yes, he was." I looked at my watch. It was time to turn around and head back. The streets were crowded as the city was waking up. I turned to Brindsley, "Breakfast time?"

He nodded and grinned.

Chapter Thirteen
Fan Fest

In two days
I get to run, The Boston Marathon
The journey has been long.
I've learned self-acceptance and love
In the miles that I've run
I will join the women before me
who gave me this opportunity.
To toe the start line
has been my dream.
I made it— thank you, team
I will race in the moment
Run, breathe, relax
I *will* be grateful for this circumstance
I know the race will hurt
I'll keep my mind alert
I've been practicing mantras in advance
To keep me calm and steady
my inner judge doesn't stand a chance
I can handle this
I have what it takes
I will endure…
 Onward!

In the days leading up to The Boston Marathon, the Boston Athletic Association set up several events for us to enjoy. They called it Fan Fest. It was held at Copley Square Park, a few blocks away from our hotel. The weekend was scheduled with live music, appearances by Boston Marathon champions, activities for the kids, and fitness classes. It was a great way to gear up for the race.

When I heard that Meb Keflezighi was going to be interviewed at Fan Fest, I was ecstatic! He was a world-class runner and four-time Olympian. He won the Boston Marathon in 2014 when the city needed a comeback from the year before. He was amazing and a hero to many of us in the running community.

When Saturday came, I made sure to arrive at Fan Fest a bit early so I could get a spot to see Meb. As I was moving through the crowd to find a spot to stand, Meb was walking my way! I couldn't believe it. I somehow found my voice. "Hi Meb!" I greeted him with a huge smile on my face. He stopped, looked at me, and said hello to me. It was incredible. *He stopped in the crowd to say hi to me.* I didn't even think he heard me. I couldn't stop smiling. He made his way to the stage and for 30 minutes he talked about his experience running The Boston Marathon, running in general, and shared some of his stories based on the questions being asked. It was inspiring. As I wiped the tears from my eyes, I noticed others were doing the same. I was grateful for this opportunity to hear him speak. It was humbling.

When he was done talking he stepped off the stage and began signing autographs, talking to runners, and taking pictures with whoever wanted one. I wanted a picture with him too. I hesitated. Jeff encouraged me to go, "Julie take my phone and get pictures, go, I'll take the kids over to the cornhole game." I joined the crowd of runners all gathered around him and waited patiently for my turn. His calm, gentle presence was contagious. He was autographing the runner's gear and clothing and agreeing to pictures.

When it was my turn, I couldn't hold back the tears. I was face-to-face with Meb! I gained my composure and somehow managed to speak the words, "May I get a picture with you?"

He said, "Yes, of course". We got several pictures together.

I thanked him for sharing his story. I wanted to say more but couldn't get the words out. He hugged me, wished me luck, and told me to stay strong. It was fantastic! (I'm tearing up just writing this.)

As I walked away to find my family, several runners gave me fist pumps and we teared up together. I had no idea how emotional this weekend was going to be. I regained my composure as I floated over to my family. I was on cloud nine. I couldn't wait to show Jeff the pictures. They were satisfied playing cornhole so I found a seat as I listened to the live music. I realized I had been on my feet all day. I sat down and took a moment to rest. *Life is good.*

I was thrilled to find out that Bill Rodgers and Amby Burfoot would be at Fan Fest on Sunday. After meeting Meb on Saturday, I couldn't believe my luck! I had no idea that racing in Boston would allow me to meet and hear from some of the world's greatest runners and people. The days leading up to the marathon were getting better and better. *How amazing is this? I didn't even run the race yet.* I was ecstatic.

Bill Rodgers and Amby Burfoot were two more running legends that I couldn't wait to see and hear from. If you aren't familiar with Bill Rodgers, let me share some of his achievements. He won four times at the Boston Marathon and four times at the New York City Marathon! When I ran collegiately, his name was brought up a lot. His name you knew as a runner, similar to Amby Burfoot. Amby Burfoot won The Boston Marathon in 1968 and, after competitive racing, he retired to become a great running journalist and author. He has published several books and his writing is encouraging and uplifting.

The fact that I would be face-to-face with Bill and Amby was inspiring! I couldn't wait to be a part of the scene. I was in Copley Square and only a few feet away from Bill and Amby. I was in awe. Being in their presence was humbling.

I made my way to the front of the crowd. Bill and Amby were all smiles as they shared their running stories and experiences. They had this energy about them that drew me in. Their laughter was contagious and all I could think as they spoke was, *I am so happy to be a runner, I am so grateful to be a part of this community.*

I loved what Amby said, "Enjoy tomorrow, slap hands, appreciate the crowd and the volunteers, thank them, and have fun. This is a celebration!"

I was happy he said this and it reminded me to place my focus here too. It took the pressure off. Yes, I wanted to run well and fast but I also wanted to remember why I ran and Amby reminded me of this. It was easy for me to forget the joy and celebration of running. The race was more than my time or place.

As I stood there listening to Amby and Bill, goosebumps covered my arms. I smiled with excitement. I was filled with gratitude for my body and mind, for running, and for the challenges I had overcome to be here. *I belonged here. I was good enough.*

I would be deliberate tomorrow to thank the volunteers, high-five the people in the crowd, encourage each runner I came in contact with on the course, and slow down a bit to celebrate. There had been many marathons in the past when this wasn't the focus. The thoughts, *You can't slow down. Don't stop. You will lose time,* controlled my focus. I would let those thoughts go and focus on what Amby said. I would have fun. I would celebrate.

Bill Rodgers' and Amby Burfoot's energy and smiles were catching. As they spoke, I felt like I already knew them, my running buddies. *Have you ever felt this before when meeting someone for the first time? It fascinates me.* I experienced this several times throughout my life. It was a great feeling. I could be myself. I belonged.

Bill leaned into the crowd as he spoke, his smile happy to see. I took a smile and a laugh for granted until those things were hidden for over a year due to COVID-19. What a difference to see a person's entire face. What a gift. I was glad we were outside where masks were not mandated. He spoke about the importance of a running buddy to keep each other going and challenge each other. I agreed. Over the last several years, especially during 2020, I was thrilled to have Felicia training with me every Saturday to keep me accountable and to support and encourage me. It made a two-hour run seem like 30 minutes as we talked about life's ups and downs, and lessons learned. She has been my consistent running buddy and has challenged me. She kept me going on days when my mind was getting in the way and I was feeling down or defeated.

I see in life and running we need each other. It's a blessing. I was happy to have found a friend who enjoyed running as much as I do. Bill and Amby mentioned that they run together often and keep each other going. Maybe that's the secret to running longevity—a great friend and running buddy. We all need someone to run alongside in life.

After Amby and Bill were done speaking, I looked at my watch. My aunt, uncle, cousin, and his family were coming to meet us. I wanted to make sure I kept my eyes open for their arrival. I couldn't wait to see them. They were making the drive from Maine. My aunt Colleen and uncle Tim were spending the night so they could watch the marathon and cheer me on. I was thrilled. My cousin, Jeremy, was making the trip over from California. I would be meeting up with him after the marathon. I was so grateful and pleased to share this moment with them and my family.

Fan Fest was crowded and I was worried we wouldn't find them, thank goodness for cell phones. My aunt called me, "We are here."

"Oh great!" and just as I said that I spotted her, my uncle, my cousin, Jed, and his family heading my way. It was great to see them and hang out with them in Boston. We walked to the finish so they could see the setup and logos painted on the street. We showed them the hotel so they knew where to meet Jeff and my mom. The hotel was just feet away from the finish line and they could all gather tomorrow. I was delighted!

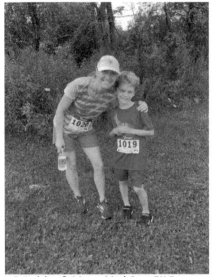

Brindsley & Me — Mad Cow 5K Race

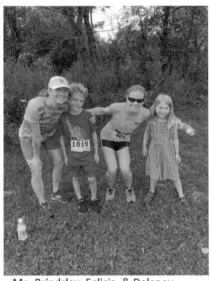

Me, Brindsley, Felicia, & Delaney

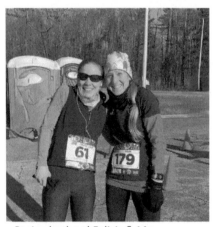

Racing back on! Felicia & Me

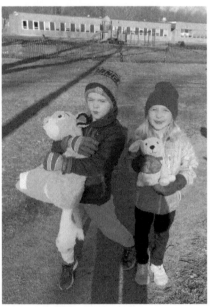

Brindsley & Delaney cheering us on.

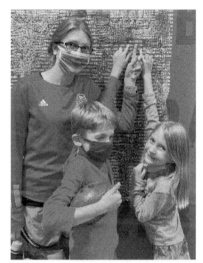

Finding my name at the Expo

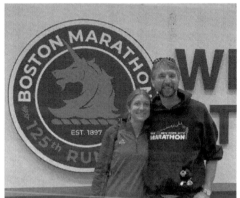

Jeff & Me at the Expo — October 8, 2021

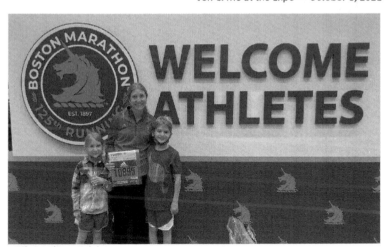

Bib number ready!

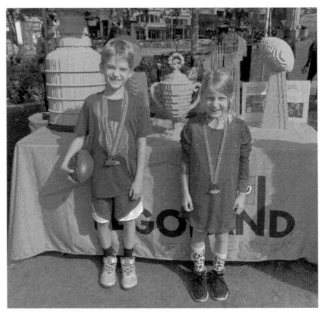

Brindsley and Delaney enjoying Fan Fest

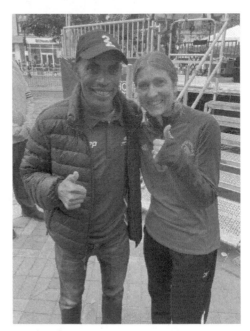

Meb Keflezighi and Me at Fan Fest —
October 9, 2021

Thrilled to meet Meb and get a picture with
him.

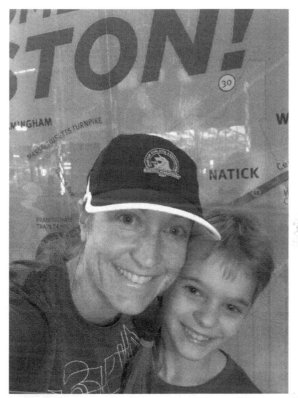

Morning run on the streets of Boston with Brindsley

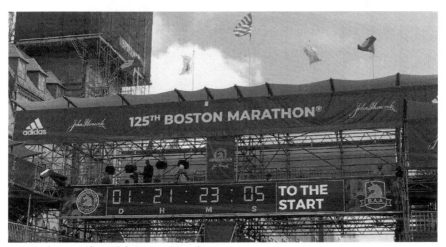

Countdown to the 125th Boston Marathon

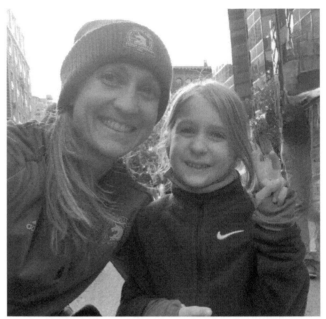

We're in BOSTON!!!

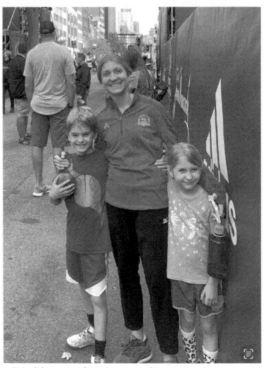

Brindsley, Me, & Delaney soaking in Boston

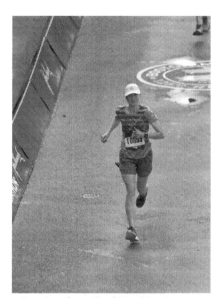

Running down Boylston Street—
Healthy, Happy, & Strong!

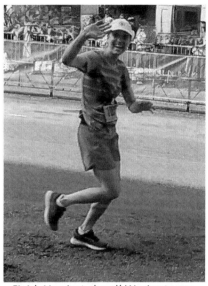

Finish Line just ahead! Waving to my
family.

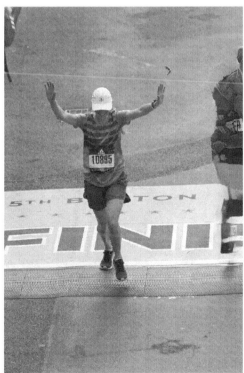

I'm a Boston Marathon Finisher!

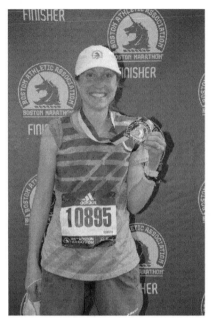

Look at the Bling!

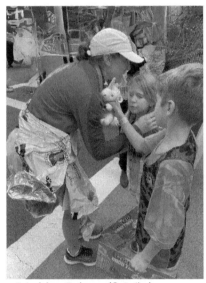

Brindsley, Delaney (& Spike)
congratulate me at the finish

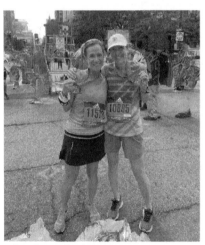

Stephanie & Me — Boston
Marathon Finishers!

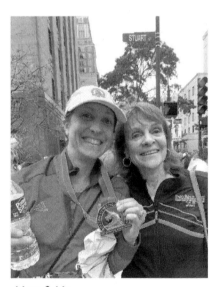

Mom & Me

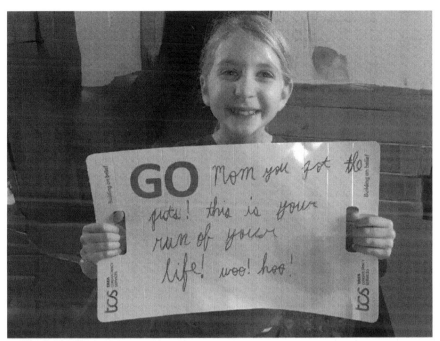

Cheer poster — Made by Delaney

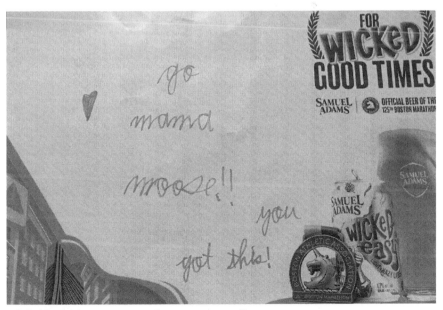

Brindsley's cheer poster — Go mama moose!!

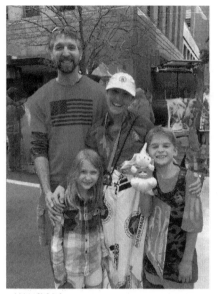

We did it!

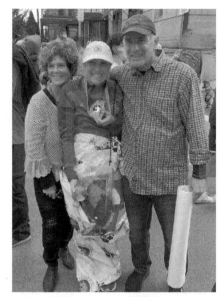

Aunt Colleen, Me, and Uncle Tim at the Finish! October 11, 2021

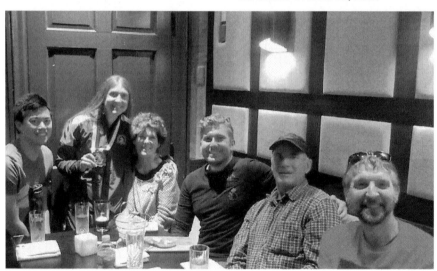

Celebrating with family

Chapter Fourteen
Shakeout

I saw a beautiful graceful willow tree
hanging down inviting me
to jump up and give it a high five
You made it to Boston
Your dream of running has come alive
I couldn't be happier
A smile across my face
Feeling connected with every runner
with each stride I make
The camaraderie is intensifying
The countdown to the marathon begins
Just like the willow tree—
Standing tall, marvelous, and strong
We are together and unified
We are Boston Strong

I hopped out of bed and tiptoed to the bathroom. Jeff and
the kids were still asleep. I changed into my running clothes
and slipped out the door. The hotel lobby was quiet with a
few guests sitting by the fireplace. I headed out of the hotel

and down the stairs to the street. *Where should I run?* I'll just head down Boylston Street.

Tomorrow was race day—time for a shakeout run. Whoever came up with the name, shakeout, was a genius. I felt like I needed to shake out the ants in my pants, the nerves, and the niggles. My right hamstring began to tingle as I started my run. *Don't freak out.* This was normal for me and my nerves were dialed up a little more than I would like. I've learned to turn my focus on what was around me—the city lights, tall buildings, and other runners striding silently down the street, loosening up before tomorrow. I heard sirens, construction work, and traffic as the city started to wake up. The tingle softened.

I continued running down Boylston street and looked to my left. It looks like a park yet as I got closer I see a sign that read Public Gardens. The massive willow trees filled the sky, and the paved trails twisted and turned throughout the Public Garden just a few blocks from my hotel. I was happy that I had chosen this direction and stumbled upon this garden. It was beautiful. This was one of the joys I find in running. Heading out the door in a new city and not knowing what you would see, hear, or find. I love exploration and because I'm on foot I could stop to take it all in or keep going. I go at my own pace. Sometimes I get turned around but I always find my way back.

I continued running in the garden and noticed the city waking up, more runners were joining me. We waved and smiled. This unspoken gift we were all anticipating was just one day away. I kept my head up and my eyes alert, I didn't want to miss a thing. The paved paths were inviting and a small stream flowed along with a bridge across it. I wanted to see more. I passed several walkers as I picked up the pace zooming around a turn.

What am I doing? I'm running too fast.

My excitement was hard to contain and I forced myself to hold back a bit. I reminded myself to slow down. Yet, I felt this energy pushing me forward and my legs moving faster with each stride. I saw a willow tree up ahead with its limbs hanging down. I felt this urge to give the willow a high five. I looked around hoping no one would see me. I jumped up to high-five the tree and then got back to running. I smiled. I was so happy to be here.

It's still early—6:30 a.m. when I finished my shakeout run. The sun was just starting to rise as I headed to the finish line, just steps away from my hotel. I stopped in front of the finish staring at the extraordinary display. The line was painted on the road in bright yellow with the words "125th Boston Marathon, FINISH," in dark blue. Before the finish line, there were several large circles on the road painted dark blue with the yellow unicorn in the center and the words "Boston Marathon, 125th Running." I stood over one with a smile.

I am here. I get to finally run this course. The thought gets louder and louder as I gazed at the finish line, the runners around me, and the countdown ticking away just above me in bright white lights.

Goosebumps covered my arms as I gaped at the lights. A portion inside me breaks free and floats upward yet I felt the ground beneath me. My spirit was celebrating this long journey and reminding me to appreciate the moment. I was cut short by the voice of another runner.

"Would you take our picture?"

I smile, "Of course. It would be my pleasure."

She handed me her phone as the two women runners huddled close over the yellow unicorn on the pavement. They beamed at the camera and were grateful for the pictures as I handed her the phone. She then offered to take a picture of me and I was ecstatic. I would love a picture and was appreciative of the gesture. I knelt on the pavement next to the large blue circle making sure the yellow unicorn was in view. I was all smiles.

Tomorrow, I will toe the start line of The Boston Marathon. My dream is coming true.

Chapter Fifteen
Eve of Boston

Boston marathon ready
Elevation gaining and steady
It's an achievable task
My mind and body I ask
Mental strength has been the focus
Mindset is what matters most, I notice
Stay brave and calm
You got this mom!
The marathon is made for you
And this I know is true
Run Brave

It was hard for me to fall asleep before a race and The Boston Marathon was no different. I laid on my back, eyes closed with my sheet pulled up to my chin. My mind recalled what I needed for tomorrow—*BIB number, drop bag, hydration, gels, and running band to carry my nutrition. Do I bring my phone? No, I'll give it to Jeff to carry. Do I have everything ready?* A mental checklist was going through my mind even though I just laid all these items out on the coffee table in the middle of the room before I went to bed.

Did I set my alarm? I leaped up in bed and grabbed my phone from the nightstand. I checked for the third time. *Yes, yes, my alarm is set.* I laid back down and laughed to myself. I recalled a few hours earlier asking the front desk for a wake-up call just in case my alarm didn't go off. *Julie, relax, you have everything set and there is nothing else you need to do. Go to sleep.*

The hotel room was quiet. Jeff and the kids were staying with my mom down the hall so I could get a good night's sleep. It felt weird not having my family with me but we thought it would be best. The last time we all stayed together the night of a race I was up a lot with the kids. My children were still at the age when interrupted sleep was a possibility. I didn't want to be up with one or both in the middle of the night. I felt bad, maybe I should've had them stay with me. *Oh! One night is fine, the decision is already made.* I resolved that thought and another creeps in preventing me from sleeping. *When should I leave to walk over to the buses to take me to the start? Should I wear a long sleeve shirt and pants on the bus or leave them in my drop bag?* Oh good Lord, all the shoulds, I guess that word was still in my vocabulary more than I would like. I pondered these questions with my eyes closed, frustrated that I was still awake. *Oh! Make sure I have a mask for the bus. I need to get to sleep.* I took some deep breaths and considered grabbing my phone to listen to a guided meditation but, as that thought entered my mind, I dozed off. The next thing I knew, the phone rang. I sat up fast and grabbed the phone.

"Hello."

"Good morning, Julie, this is your wake-up call."

"Oh thank you, that came quickly."

I hung up the phone and I was out of bed ready to go. It was nice to turn the lights on and not tip-toe around in the dark. I jumped in the shower repeating my mantras and what I would say when the going gets tough. I put on my watch next to my LIVESTRONG bracelet. I'd worn this bracelet since 2011 when Jeff was diagnosed with testicular cancer. It was a reminder to me of the challenges we had overcome together and to stay strong when times were tough. I was amazed at how durable the bracelet was. I've had it on for ten years.

I head to the coffee table in the middle of the room where I laid out my clothes. I get dressed and then make my breakfast. I brought my toaster for my gluten-free bread. I spread a little almond butter and sliced bananas on top of the bread. I grabbed a water bottle from the refrigerator and started taking sips. The weather was going to be nice although a bit on the warm side for a marathon. I wanted to make sure I stayed ahead on my hydration. I began packing my clear plastic bag with a few items that I wanted after the race — warm clothes, a water bottle, and some food.

I was finishing up when Jeff came in. "Hey Jules, how did you sleep?"

"Well, good I guess. It just took me a while to fall asleep. How did you and the kids do?"

"We slept okay, they are already up. Are you ready? I'll walk you to the buses."

"Oh good, I would love that."

I grabbed my bag and gave my phone to Jeff in case anyone called. I didn't want to carry my phone with me. We walked down the hall to see Brindsley, Delaney, and my mom before I headed to the buses. It was so great to see them, and I could tell that the kids were excited to be with Nana. I hugged them all, and my mom took a few pictures.

"Thank you mom for being here, it means a lot."

"Julie, I'm so glad to be here and to help out."

I was blessed to have my mom still around and glad she was healthy to keep up with my children.

Jeff and I put on our masks and took the next elevator down to the lobby. When we stepped out, I was surprised by crowds of runners making their way to the buses too. We all gathered together as we made our way down Boylston Street and past Copley Square to the Public Gardens where the buses were lined up. I stopped to drop my bag off and then said goodbye to Jeff. We hugged as he whispered, "Good luck honey, and have fun!" I hugged him tight and thanked him for his support and encouragement all these years. I held back tears as I weaved around runners to get in line for the bus. There were people everywhere and we were all huddled together waiting for the next load of buses.

"Here they come!" I heard a voice shout as we watched them line up in front of us. A volunteer instructed us to get on any bus that wasn't full and reminded us all to wear a mask. I began walking towards the buses wondering which one to get on. I picked the third bus from the front. I wish I had picked the first or even the second bus— *hindsight is always 20/20.*

Chapter Sixteen
Unexpected Detour

My mind is on the run.
I feel tense— swallowed up
by my sentences. I turn the
corner, and the wind whispers
in my ear— *Listen.*

The stream roars
drowns out my commotion.
My arms glide and float with
each stride. The wind whispers
in my ear— *Look.*

A hawk soars, an effortless
flight high above the tree line.
My body softens. I lean in drift
among the trail. My mind is like
a pond with no ripples.

Strength from the wind,
calm from the water.
Peace returns.

Oh no! We are lost! I'm not going to get to the start. I'm not going to get to run Boston.

My mind immediately thought the worst. I was upset and nervous. I ruminated on what I could have done differently like I was supposed to know the bus driver was going to get lost. I'd been waiting for over 20 years to toe this start line. Didn't the bus driver know?

Of course, something like this would happen.

I felt in-between emotions of laughter and tears. This was life. We go in with a plan, exactly what we want and what needs to happen and it would many times go sideways. I'd liked to think I was a veteran at this. You know the song — "You can't always get what you want?" I'd learned that over the years. *But God has a plan and purpose. This marathon, the one I'm racing today, I vowed to run in 2003.* Yet God knew it wasn't the time for me. I wasn't healthy and He intervened.

It has been a process to get here and as I sat on the bus I had time to reflect on it.

Maybe that's why the bus driver is lost. Let's look at the silver lining Julie. When we look for it we will find it and it's a better option than getting my panties all in a bunch. This was a trivial matter, we would get to the race just maybe not how or when I expected.

Life was full of unexpected detours, and how I responded was what mattered. I took some deep breaths.

Julie relax. Don't freak out. You will get to the race today. You will be right on time. I repeated this sentence though it wasn't convincing. *Ugh, I can't believe this is happening.* There I go again… right back to the negative. I looked out the window trying to focus on something else. Something to shift my mindset.

Look at the trees. Oh yes, the red and orange leaves were gorgeous.

This distracted me for about a second then my mind was racing again. *What kind of bus driver doesn't know how to get to the start line? Didn't they practice the route?* I was on fire with anger when we came to a stop. *What's going on?* I craned my head over the seat in front of me and peeked over. Through the bus window, I spotted a cop car blocking the road. *He has to let us through. We are all runners. We need to get to the start.* The cop walked over to the bus and the bus driver opened his doors. I was unable to hear what he was saying to the bus driver.

A runner got off the bus, he needed to use the bathroom. A few runners ahead of me shouted, "We need to get off this bus. The cop is not going to let us through. Do you trust this guy getting us to the start line? He is lost!"

I panicked. *What should I do? I better get off too.* We could walk and find our way to the start. I stood up and saw runners starting to head off the bus. *I better go with them.* I figured it was better to be with a group to find our way together. I looked at my bus seat buddy and told her I was getting off. I slipped past her and joined the line of runners making their way off the bus. I stepped off the bus, my stomach flip-flopping at what had just occurred. I felt like I was going to throw up. *Julie, keep it together.*

I started speed walking with the rest of my bus buddies. I was glad to take my mask off. I didn't look behind me but heard there were three other buses behind ours, they were following us. *That stinks.* I wonder if they would walk too or stay on the bus. We had a two-mile walk according to one of the runners who pulled up the directions on his phone. *Thank goodness I'm with someone who has a phone.* I continued to talk to myself. *I'm doing the right thing. Focus on my mind-set. Don't let this walk uphill deter my race. Julie, keep a good attitude. This will be a great warm-up.*

This was not in the plan yet I refused to let this ruin my first Boston Marathon experience. Another runner caught up to our group, "Well, I guess if we can run 26.2 miles we can certainly walk two miles before we start." She was right, what were two more miles? I didn't need to make this mean it would affect my race negatively though that's exactly where my inner judge was taking me. *Why didn't you stay on the bus with the driver?* Oh Aunt Phoebe, you rascal! I refused to spiral and let the negative thoughts win. I'd been working so hard on this, to manage my mind and pivot. If there was one thing I improved on in 2020 it was this! Instead of freaking out like the old Julie would have done, I smiled and laughed with the others walking with me.

I will get to the start. I'm not alone. I repeated these sentences to stay calm and optimistic. *I am in great company. We are in this together. I will race The Boston Marathon today!* The best part of this year was a rolling start. Once we arrived at the start area we would be able to hydrate, use the bathroom, warm-up, and then start when we were ready. We would be right on time and that thought was worth repeating. *I will be right on time.*

I looked to my right, and a few runners hustled with me, their determined eyes focused straight ahead as we approached a hill. One shouted, "Well, we'll have something to talk about, won't we?" I leaned forward and announced, "I'm going to write a book about this." We all grinned at each other as we continued the climb.

A few spectators were heading our way. They looked at us with confused faces as our bib numbers were visible and we collectively shouted, "The bus got lost!"

They shouted back, "Keep going straight. You are almost there!"

We all breathed a sigh of relief, "Thank you!" Any anxiety or doubt we were carrying was now washed away with calm and certainty. We were almost there. We were not lost.

The bright colors of the leaves on our right and left surrounded us as we dashed up the hill. I began to hear cheers and shouts in the distance. We must be close yet we had no idea where the start line was. We crested the top of the hill. I looked up to a sea of heads bobbing, runners with bib numbers covering the road, spectators and volunteers in all directions, and a booming voice over the loudspeaker. My jaw dropped open in awe as I gazed at my surroundings.

The road was blocked off by barriers. Several cops and volunteers were standing at the ready. They saw us jogging towards them and one walked to meet us. In unison, we blurted out, "The bus got lost!" Before she let us through, she checked for our bib numbers and bracelets. "Good luck!" she shouted as we rushed past her.

We made it! This is the start of the 125th Boston Marathon.

Chapter Seventeen
Breathe, Relax, and Run

Toe the start line— racers set
Gather together, elbow to elbow
like we've already met.

The horn sounds, and off we go!
A stream of color—
Legs and arms flow.

Spectators line the roads
Cheers give goosebumps to
our toes.

Sunshine beats down on the trees
Beautiful fall painting
for us to see.

Appreciation and smiles
for our body and mind—
as we cross the finish line.

My arms and legs tingled with excitement. I stood still for a moment, my blue running sneakers glued to the black pavement, taking in the scene. I was awestruck. I didn't want to forget this.

I'm here! I made it!

I wanted to shout but my voice was stuck in my throat. An image of me running through the crowd high-fiving and hugging every runner flashed in my mind. It didn't seem all that crazy as tears started to well up. I turned my head towards the voice of the announcer—the start line! There it was. A crowd of spectators on each side of the road sent prickles down my spine as their cheers filled my ears. I took a deep breath and gathered myself. This tremendous feeling of appreciation, gratitude, and belonging covered me. I tried to shove these feelings down, push them away, and act like I'd been here before, yet my body and mind knew the truth. This was the marathon we had been training for. This was the long-awaited dream coming to fruition. The years of training, of setbacks, of trying again, and trying again, were finally here.

Let's go, Julie.

I regained my focus. My eyes quickly scanned for the nearest volunteer to guide me to the porta-potties. I could feel my body beginning to tense up, my anxiety getting the best of me. The two-mile walk to the start was not what I had planned or expected. I looked down at my watch, I'm here at the start 40 minutes later. I walked past runners heading to the start line and my nerves buzzed with a mix of excitement, anxiety, and apprehension. In this state, I tend to talk very fast, my mind three steps ahead of my body, and I forget to breathe. Luckily, the volunteer was clear and kind, helping me with the questions I was spitting out at her. *Where are the closest porta-potties? Where do I go? How do I get to the start line? Do I just jump in with the runners to get to the start line? The bus got lost so I'm not sure what's going on.*

She was so calm and patient with me. She smiled at me as she answered my questions. I was happy she chose not to wear a mask outside. Her smile was exactly what I needed, my reminder to breathe, relax, and stay calm. She instructed me to give her any clothes I didn't want to run in. I began taking off my sweatpants and long sleeve shirt. It was getting warm already. She shoved them in the plastic bag she was holding and pointed up the incline to where the porta-potties were. "They are just up ahead to your right. You can't miss them. All the runners will be there. Have fun."

I jogged up to the porta-potties, all lined up bright blue with white-covered tops. Hundreds of runners swarmed in and out of each one. I scanned the lines trying to find the shortest. Runners were sitting on the ground stretching, some standing and chatting, and the rest in line for the bathroom. It was chaos and wild. Just a year ago this was not even possible because of COVID. It was hard to believe we were finally here. The energy was contagious and as I waited, the music, announcer, and spectators' shouts all filled the air. I tried to take it all in. This was part of the racing that I missed. The chaos, crowds, cheering, and excited people were everywhere. We were all here to run the same distance and course— it was incredible. I looked at my watch, it was 10:35 a.m. I wanted to start at 10:15 a.m. *Oh well, take a breath Julie, it's a rolling start. You are right on time.* That thought relaxed me as I waited in line for the bathroom. Runners were all around me, laughing, smiling, and talking. It was incredible to be around so many people again and racing. It was fantastic to be back in this atmosphere. There wasn't anything like it. *Today I will race the Boston Marathon, bring a good attitude, and enjoy this day. I got this. Breathe, relax, run. Breathe, relax, run.*

As I waited for my turn, I double-checked that my sneakers were tied well and my BIB number was fastened and visible. I stood there overhearing a conversation behind me, between two women runners. Their conversation went something like this, "I'm just here to run and have fun, but I'm still so nervous." "I know me too, I have run this so many times, but I still am worried about my time, I just want to have fun and celebrate being back here."

I could resonate with their conversation. I was feeling similar—the nervous feeling, worry, and the drive to run well yet have fun. I'm sure many other runners felt the same. We all had our own stories that got us here yet we all hoped to enjoy ourselves and do well. I thought about what this meant for me. *What does that look like for me?* Running well, yet having fun, and being happy I'm here. I promised myself that whatever time I saw on my watch, I wouldn't beat myself up and I would be grateful. This wasn't easy to do. My old story of perfection and performance had been ingrained in me yet over the years, with help from God, I've confronted this. Thankfully God's love was not based on performance or ability. My self-worth was not based on appearance, performance, or pleasing others.

I know the truth and the truth will set you free. The joy of running has come back to me.

Chapter Eighteen
The Dream

The dream began in 1998
to run The Boston Marathon
was going to be great.
I was eager in 2003, yet my
body and mind didn't agree.
The pain took over
and consumed my days.
I wanted to keep running—
push through, shove it down
I believed that was the way.

God had a plan—I'd have to wait.
Shame rooted deep, an inside job
I would need to reap. Face my fears,
do not hide. He gave me strength and
never left my side.

To follow my dream I would need to let go.
The burdens I was carrying, too many,
I know. Conformed by thoughts
no longer true. It's okay to question—
start a new.

I held tight to Courage and began to unpack.
My load getting lighter as my runs
were coming back. I don't need fixing after all.
Everything was already inside me—
My focus returned to the Lord to guide me.

The Boston Marathon had been on my mind since 1998 after I finished my first marathon as a high school senior. Yes, I was that crazy human who crossed the finish line exhausted and uncomfortable, yet ready to do it all over again. *Sign me up! When's the next marathon?*

I had no idea it would take over 20 years to toe The Boston Marathon line—but God knew. The setbacks, try-again, and challenges—God was working through it all. *Keep fighting Julie. Keep pressing on!* I finally asked God for help and He never left my side. I made it. Tears filled my eyes as I made my way to the start line. *This is happening?* I wanted to pinch myself to make sure it wasn't a dream. I weaved around runners. Upbeat music filled our ears as we smiled at one another. *Today we run the freaking Boston Marathon.* I crossed over the start line and started my watch. My race has begun. The cheers and shouts sent a flood of adrenaline through my legs—I was sprinting at the start of the race. I looked to my left and saw runners walking on the side of the road heading in the direction I just came from. *That must be an-other bus of runners that got lost.* I felt bad that so many of us didn't get to the right location. I turned my attention back to the race. I needed to pace myself during the first half by not going too fast. I had heard this from so many veterans who had finished this marathon. Gosh was it hard not to take off at a fast pace. We were heading downhill and the adrenaline from the excitement was overwhelming. There were so many downhills that made it hard for me to slow down. Runners surrounded me and we all seemed to be in unison—*we need to pace ourselves.* I was happy that the running band was working out well and not bouncing around. I felt a bit lighter without the vest and was confident this would work. At mile two, I reached back and grabbed one of the soft flasks of fluid. I remembered what Joel said, "Take fluids early and often. Don't get behind in your hydration and nutrition." I took a few sips and then reached behind to put it back in the waistband pouch. I dropped it. A runner behind shouted, "You dropped your bottle". I stopped and turned around to pick it up, thanking him as I grabbed it off the concrete. I was a bit upset that I had dropped it. Yet, I was not used to reaching behind to grab my hydration, I'd practiced with it always in a vest in front of me. *Julie, you will need to be a bit more mindful of this. You don't want to lose your hydration in the beginning miles.* I shoved it back in to make sure the other one was in there too and both were secure. *Ugh, I probably just lost two minutes turning around to pick that up.*

No. Julie, you are good. Take a breath and relax. It's okay. You got this. I made sure to redirect my thinking immediately, it was way too early in the race to beat myself up, and I wouldn't allow it. I promised myself no matter what happened that I was to talk kindly to myself.

I'm going too fast! Dang, now I'm going too slow... ugh... pace yourself, Julie! I can't go too fast or I won't make it up Heartbreak Hill!

This was my inner dialogue for the first five miles of The Boston Marathon. NOT helpful or what I had planned to be thinking on. I kept looking down at my watch. I couldn't get a consistent pace. My worry and anxiety were both starting to take over. My self-talk wasn't helpful. I know that beating myself up only hinders my performance. And I was only at mile five. I had 21.2 miles to go! I had to change something.

I stopped looking down at my watch. I stopped beating myself up. I looked up and around instead. *Hello Boston Marathon! I'm running the freaking Boston Marathon! WOOHOO!* A huge grin came to my face, and I said it again to myself. *I'm running the freaking Boston Marathon!* I got goosebumps as I repeated it. The goosebumps multiplied as hundreds of spectators lined up on each side of the road to cheer us on. Crazy signs that read, "Don't trust a fart" and "You thought it said 'rum' didn't you," made me laugh. Children were lined up with high-fives and fist pumps, and music blasted from random homes as we pressed on. It was amazing. And just like that my thoughts were back on track.

I began repeating, *Breathe, relax, run. Breathe, relax, run.* I took it all in and was in awe that I was a part of this marathon.

It was more than I could ever imagine or read about. Yet, this was why The Boston Marathon was my dream. This was why I never gave up.

I no longer thought about my pace or strategy. I knew I would finish. I thought about Bobbi Gibb and Kathrine Switzer. It was an overwhelming feeling of pride, appreciation, and gratitude. My time didn't matter. My place didn't matter. I was here. *Julie, take it all in—celebrate this moment that took so many years to achieve.*

***

At mile 13 the ache and burning sensation in my legs got louder. My body caught on that we were still running. My thoughts started to focus on the discomfort and the fatigue. The spiral that I knew I had to fight was suddenly shut down by the overwhelming screams filling my ears.

I looked to my right—hundreds of screaming spectators were jumping up and down holding signs. A warm shiver covered my body as I realized where I was. I made it to Wellesley College, the halfway mark of The Boston Marathon. They called it the Scream Tunnel. The videos I watched and the books I read on this part of the race couldn't have prepared me for the REAL live experience.

My smile lit up the Scream Tunnel. I couldn't help but pick up the pace. I was floating, this out-of-body experience as I coast past. I wanted to slow down, read every sign, and slap every hand, yet my legs were flying. I couldn't stop. The screams of encouragement were following me as I continued ahead and the discomfort disappeared. I was running The Boston Marathon. My desire to be present and be in the moment returned. *I am here.*

I continued to coach myself through the miles ahead. It was getting warm and I was out of the hydration that I was carrying. I was glad to have the volunteers every mile handing out water and Gatorade. I grabbed both. I didn't want to get behind on my hydration. I was witnessing many runners cramping up. One runner behind me yelled up to his friend, "Hey Joe, my calf is cramping up. I gotta stop for a bit." My thoughts switched from worry about the pace to hydration to Joe's friend—*I hope he is okay and can keep going.*

I better start drinking every mile until the end. I wanted to do all I could to prevent that from happening to me. Even with all the hydration I was consuming, I was so thirsty. Just when I started to spiral down with the thought of *I'm so hot, and I hope I don't cramp up,* a wonderful thing happened… sponges! Yet not just any sponges… an ice-cold blue and yellow square squish of refreshment. *The joy of looking up!*

Several women were standing on the right side of the road handing out these sponges full of water. It was a miracle. I weaved between several runners to make my way over to them. I grabbed one as I shouted, "Thank you!" I squeezed the bright blue sponge all over the front and back of my neck. It was glorious! The sponge was so cool it surprised me. *How did they get them so cold? Wow, this feels great! Thank you, Lord!* I was so grateful and happy for that one blue and yellow square sponge.

The ice-cold water that came out of that one tiny sponge was shocking! It cooled me right down and the thought of being so hot was gone. I was energized and relieved. What a generous and loving thing to do for us. I noticed and was aware of this outpouring of love and generosity all along the road to Boston. It was beautiful. The goosebumps returned as I looked around at what I was a part of. Thousands of marathoners running ahead of me, alongside me, and behind me. We were running the roads from Hopkinton to Boston. We were in this together. *I got this. I can do this.*

That one sponge was a turning point for me in the race. My negative self-talk was drowned out again by the cheers and shouts of the crowd as I began my climb. The famous Heartbreak Hill was here. I was determined to not back down. I could see several runners walking and I was fighting back the urge to do the same. My mantra of—*My legs are strong. I've trained for this. I have what it takes* was my thought loop as I began to ascend Heartbreak Hill.

Chapter Nineteen
Heartbreak Hill

They call it Heartbreak Hill
And now I know why
It's perfectly placed in the marathon
To make you dig deep—
It may even make you weep.

The yells and shouts from the crowd
Keep you going and feeling proud
Your legs want to slow down
but your mind says NO!
Let's Go, don't stop
You're almost to the top
Don't back down
Pump your arms, shorten your stride
Lean forward, and enjoy the ride.

It will be hard
It will be tough
You will make it to the top
Don't stop!

Your dream coming true
As you take in the view
You feel a pull
It's your heart not breaking
But full.

Heartbreak Hill will test you mentally and physically.

I'd read many books about this marathon and knew this was the spot, the moment in the race that would test me. I faced a steep half-mile uphill run. I was at mile 20.

What will I say to myself to keep going? How will I convince my body and mind that the fatigue, pain, and burning are worth it?

I leaned forward and pumped my arms with all my might yet my legs were heavy. I felt like a snail inching along the road—*Am I even moving forward?* The burning sensation in my thighs and calves was getting louder. My mind screamed at me to stop. Then the best thing happened, a man shouted, "Keep pumping your arms and drive those knees. You got this hill!" I felt like he was talking directly to me and I listened. I didn't give up on my body. I continued to pump my arms and trusted that my legs would get me up the hill or what felt more like a mountain.

My mantra returned—*My legs are strong. I have what it takes, and this is temporary.* I repeated this sentence one more time then it was drowned out by the cheers and shouts of the spectators covering Heartbreak Hill. They picked me up just when I needed it and my focus shifted to their cheers and shouts of encouragement.

It was at this moment I wanted to stop and tell every spectator how much they meant to me. The joy of the cheers! Thank you. *Your cheers are a blessing. You are a blessing! You are helping us more than you know. Your support, crazy signs, bell ringing, high fives, and shouts matter! You matter.*

I pressed on reminding myself this discomfort was temporary. The burning, aching, and fatigue would all go away once I crossed the finish line. I welcomed the burning sensation and accepted it. I was running up Heartbreak Hill! You betcha I would feel the burn and hurt. I didn't need to stop though, the sooner I made it up the better. I recalled all the hills I trained on to get to this point. I got this as I looked up to see more uphill coming at me. *Yikes, there's more!*

I took a deep breath and shook out my arms. *Okay, let's go!* I began giving myself a pep talk to get up what seemed to be the unceasing Heartbreak Hill. Yet, I was happy about it. Even though I was hurting, I was grateful to be making this climb. Heartbreak Hill forced me to slow down, to consciously choose to be present, to keep looking up, and to take in the love and generosity of others. Appreciate and celebrate this experience. It took me so long to get here yet it would be over soon. The marathon and the goal that I'd been working towards for so many years would end. *Once I crest this hill I only have five miles to go.* I wished for more miles, more miles to cherish this achievement. I knew that sounded crazy yet, as I made my way to the crest of Heartbreak Hill, I wanted to turn around and start again. I didn't want the marathon to end.

The burning sensation in my thighs and calf muscles was hard to block out. I was running up Heartbreak Hill — "The Mountain" as I have read the Kenyans refer to it. It certainly did feel like a mountain. *Keep moving my legs. Don't stop.* My mantra continued. *My legs are strong, I have what it takes.* I refused to walk though I wondered if I walked would I make it up the hill faster? I questioned this as yet another runner started walking. As I looked up to see more uphill coming at me, I wondered if maybe they knew something I didn't.

Heartbreak Hill kept going. It seemed like it was miles. I felt there was one steady incline, a small break then another steady incline. Whether this was actually what it was like or just my eyes playing tricks on me I can't say, but mentally maybe it helped me think about it in this way to tackle it in bits. I pumped my arms harder hoping that would speed up my legs. I didn't feel like I was running very fast. *I gotta get going. Come on Julie pick up the pace. You can do it.* I gave myself a pep talk on the last steady incline and now I was at mile 21. *Okay, five more miles to go. Give it all you got.* My legs were tired but my thoughts surprisingly gave me another spurt of energy, and I felt like I was picking up the pace. I didn't bother looking down at my watch. I continued looking up. *How many runners can I catch?* This was the game I played with five miles to go. I felt like this helped my brain focus on that instead of the fatigue, aches, and discomfort.

Wait! I only have five miles left to go and I'm not having any nerve symptoms. In the last marathon, just a year ago, I had nerve pain in my right hip down to my knee and into my right calf muscle. Today, nothing and it wakes me up a bit to push harder. *Julie, no nerve symptoms. Get moving.* Yes, my legs were tired and sore and burning but no nerve tingling, numbness, or weird sharp stabs. None of it. It was a miracle for me! I had those symptoms for over the last ten years, and when I ran marathons, I had to learn to manage those symptoms. Today, I didn't.

As I kept going I was in awe of all the spectators, constant cheers, and signs being held up all along the streets. *Oh my gosh! This is amazing!* And then there it was… the CITGO sign! This sign has had a historic presence along the race route. It was letting me know that I was one mile from the finish. I never thought I would be so happy to see that sign. I was almost there. Seeing CITGO was my reassurance and confirmation that I would finish The Boston Marathon. I was going to cross the line of the most prestigious marathon in the world. As I got closer and closer to Boylston Street, my mind turned to my family. The streets were packed with spectators on both sides. *I hope I will be able to see them before I cross the finish line. I hope the Boston app that Jeff had on his phone was letting them know my location.*

I turned onto Boylston Street and was running head-on into a wall of cheers, shouts, people jumping up and down, signs, and the ringing of cowbells. The hair on my arms was standing on end. I kept my eyes ahead and I saw the finish line in the distance. I was overcome with joy. I whispered through misty eyes, *I made it. I'm going to cross the finish.*

I pushed through the burning and fatigue in my muscles as I kept my eyes on the finish line now blurry from my tears. I was almost there. I glanced over to the right every couple of strides in hopes of seeing my family standing there. The sound of my breathing was muffled by the cowbells ringing, the announcer over the loudspeaker, and the tremendous cheers from both sides of the street. *WOW!* The feeling of awe consumed me with goosebumps to prove it. I felt this warm fuzzy sensation all over my body. *What was this?* This was joy, happiness, and accomplishment. This was how it showed up for me and I was noticing it. I was grateful. What a wonderful feeling as I coasted closer to the finish line.

I scanned the crowd and still didn't see anyone. I brought my attention back to the finish line and saw a runner 100 feet ahead collapse. *Oh my gosh, I need to help him.* But then I hear "JULIE! JULIE!" My eyes darted to the right to find Jeff shouting my name and waving. I noticed three other runners carrying the runner who fell to the finish. My mom, children, Aunt Colleen, and Uncle Tim were all there with Jeff cheering for me. I found them. My grin was as wide as the street as I gave them a wave. My children's faces lit up as they jumped up and down with their signs. They were hanging over the guardrails shouting "GO, MAMA!" A surge of energy from the sound of their voices took over my legs as I picked up the pace. My arms were raised in celebration as I crossed the thick yellow paint on the road with the blue letters reading "FINISHER." I had raced and finished the 125th Boston Marathon.

Chapter Twenty
Running is Connection

Running is solitude
Running is space
Running is breathe, relax
Keep my pace.

Running is to fly
Running is free
Running is uphill and down
A time to be me.

Running is exploration
Running is release
Running is meditative
Settle in and be.

Running is conversation
Running is play
Running is joy and love
Fresh air, yay!

Sweat and tears covered my eyes, cheeks, and chin as I crossed over the finish line. My legs were mush under my body but I didn't want to sit down. I forced myself to stand tall and look out over the finish. I smiled. I stared at the bold yellow finish line, the brave runners making their last strides to the finish, and scanned the crowd of spectators cheering and clapping for us all. I observed the volunteers guiding, supporting, and assisting anyone who was in need. They were handing out disposable masks at the finish if you wanted one. I wanted to take it all in.

We did it! I did it!

I'm in awe of what I just accomplished—I wanted to pinch myself. *Did I just run The Boston Marathon?* My entire body shouted YES! I was hurting. I was tired. My muscles were burning but I couldn't stop smiling. It was hard not to limp. My right hip nudged me to start moving. I moved slowly toward the volunteer who handed me a bottle of water. I took a few sips. I didn't want to leave. My feet stuck to the road as other runners walked past me. I was in a daze. *Was this a dream?* I closed my eyes and listened. I heard cheers, clapping, and cowbells ringing from the crowd. I heard the announcer calling out names of runners who were, now Boston Marathon finishers. I didn't want to forget this day. I wanted it ingrained in my mind. I wanted this memory to be stamped in my brain so I could easily access it whenever I needed a reminder of what I was capable of, of what my mind and body were capable of. Thank you, Lord. Nothing was impossible with Him.

Why do we forget? Why do we let our minds run to doubt, judgment, or criticism? Why do we let the enemy take a seat, steal our joy, and tell us we are not worthy? It's a daily fight for me. I have to kick the enemy out every day. That's the truth. It's a real struggle some days yet I've seen what God can do. He is always working and making a way. He is good. And He is why I'm even here today to write this story. He made a way for me. He placed the people in my life to guide and coach me.

I stopped and looked around. We all just ran The Boston Marathon. My dream came true from the first marathon I ran in 1998 to honor my teammate who died of leukemia to now, 2021. What a humbling journey.

***

I began limping toward the volunteers handing out the medals. A concerned marathoner approached me, "Are you okay? Do you need a shoulder?" She walked up next to me. She was wearing a bright yellow shirt, black shorts, and bright pink sneakers. Her kind face and smile made me think we had met before.

"Do you need to go to the medical tent?" she asked. I guess my limping was obvious.

"No, really, I'm fine. Thank you so much, but I'll just take your shoulder." I placed my hand on her shoulder as we both walked, heads held high, to grab our medals. Her name was Stephanie and she was from San Antonio, Texas.

This was her second Boston Marathon, counting the virtual as her first. It was the same for me and we were both glowing as we talked about the experience.

She lifted her elbow, it was bleeding and scraped up. "Oh my gosh, what happened?" I asked concerned. "I fell. I tripped on a bump in the road and landed in front of a police officer. The officer said it was the most graceful fall she has ever seen," she shrugged and smiled.

We both laughed as we stopped to grab our medals. Our eyes lit up as we placed the gold unicorn medal over our heads. She had her phone and snapped some pictures of us together like we were old friends. It was such a joy to meet her. I gave her my number so she could send me the pictures. We waved goodbye and congratulated each other. We hoped to stay in touch and see each other again in Boston.

I believe this was one reason runners come back. It's the friends we meet, the connections we make. This city welcomes you with open arms and you feel the energy, the excitement all around you. Who doesn't want to experience that?

I turned the corner to find my family, slowing down to watch, listen, and take in the atmosphere. Hundreds of people gathered on the roads as I weaved around smiles, laughter, and pictures being taken. It was incredible to see. It was almost like the dream I had several nights ago. Yet this wasn't a dream. It was real. As I moved through the crowd my eyes scanned ahead, and I spotted a familiar face. *My mom! There's my family.* I smiled as tears filled my eyes. My mom hugged me. I whispered, "I did it, mom. I finally did it."

She replied, "Yes you did. You did amazing, Julie. Your dream came true."

My children raced up to me smiling wide and shouting "MAMA, MOM, look at our signs!"

"Yes, please! I want to see those signs after I give you a sweaty hug and kiss."

My children proudly held them up for me to read.

Brindsley wrote, "Go mama moose you got this!" I had no idea how that nickname came to be. Delaney's poster read "Mom, you got the guts, you are running the race of your life. You can do it 2021!! Goooo, mom!"

Tears touched my eyes. My children were a blessing.

Jeff came over to congratulate me with open arms. "Jules, you did great", as he pulled me in for a hug. "This marathon is amazing. You have to see the finish from the hotel." I was so happy to see him so excited about a marathon. I was grateful for his support and encouragement over these last five years. My aunt and uncle came over with a cheer sign and smiled. I hugged them both, grateful they made the trip to cheer me on. My aunt and uncle have been so supportive over the years and my uncles' positive influence on me as a child was a big reason I turned to running. I couldn't thank him enough for introducing me to road races and track clubs when I was young.

I felt this tremendous gratitude and appreciation for my family and friends' support and encouragement. My cousins made the trip to see me and congratulated me. I had many text messages and emails before and after the race—I felt so much love. It was hard for me to communicate in words how amazing this moment felt. I hope my family and friends know how much I love and appreciate them. I hope they know how much they mean to me.

***

We stood on the corner of Stuart Street taking pictures and enjoying the atmosphere. My children were excited to see the medal, the new bling for them to try on. Delaney placed it over her head. "Look at me, mom!"

Then Brindsley gave it a try announcing, "I'm going to run this marathon too."

I was so excited to see them and wanted to know all about their morning. The concerned mother in me began shooting off questions, "Jeff did everything go okay? Did you end up staying at the hotel or walking around? How were the kids? Did they behave okay for my mom?" I was so eager to find out what they were doing while I was running. They were thrilled to tell me about their epic breakfast and a TV show they watched in Nana's hotel room.

"Mom, we watched Trolls, it's the best show ever."

I laughed and maybe you are too. *Yes, my kids just watched Trolls for the first time and it's 2021.*

They filled me in on the rest of their morning and how exciting it was to see all the runners finishing. In all the excitement, I didn't mention the bus getting lost and my long walk to find the start line. However, at that moment Jeff inquired, "You started the race later than you planned."

"Oh gosh, I sure did. I have a story to tell you. You won't believe what happened. Remind me when we sit down and eat. I'll tell you then." I was curious how my aunt and uncle made out finding Jeff and my mom. "It all worked out great!" my aunt smiled. "We met your mom in the lobby and got the okay from the hotel staff to view the marathon with them." Oh great! I was so happy everything worked out so well.

I couldn't stop smiling and congratulating all the runners as we walked back to the hotel. It was amazing. There was not one person without a smile on their face. I could still hear the cheers as marathoners were finishing. "Jeff, I gotta check out the finish."

My mom took the kids back to her room so Jeff and I could hang out at the finish. It was awesome to be on the other side, to be cheering and shouting as I knew how much it mattered. I wanted to jump in and run to experience the finish again. I think Jeff could read my mind, as he turned to me and said, "We gotta come back here again. This marathon is awesome."

I smiled, "Absolutely, we are coming back, I want to run this again." We made our way back to the hotel to get cleaned up.

As I entered the hotel, a line of employees were standing in the foyer clapping and congratulating me. They were all wearing blue t-shirts that read "Run Boston" on the front. I was so surprised. I stood there thanking them with tears in my eyes. I felt like I was in a dream. *Was this really happening?* I guess it was kind of hard to hide this unicorn medal around my neck or the light shining from my head to the tips of my toes. *You will glow after you cross the finish line of The Boston Marathon.* They were right. I was glowing.

Chapter Twenty-One
Thank You Body

Thank you body
for the miles I get
to run— my time to reflect
on all my body has done.

Thank you body
for my powerful legs
just what I need to
make the elevation gains.

Thank you body
Working for me
Even when I treated
you very poorly.

Thank you body
for letting me know
I'm so thrilled we have
more years to go.

Thank you body
I'm listening to you
I feel healthy, happy, and strong

I've changed my point of view.

I was so happy that I finished that I'd forgotten about the soreness and discomfort in my legs until I stepped into the shower. *Oh! I am sore.* I stood under the warm water to relax but not for long. "Ouch," I shouted as the water stung and burned the inner part of my legs. It was painful.

Jeff yelled in, "Are you okay?" I was clenching and cringing as the water splashed down. I had no idea about the chafing I had until the water hit my skin. I got out of the shower quickly, holding back tears.

My skin was so raw and red. I yelled out to him, "I'm chafed bad. Does anyone have any vaseline or lotion?" Jeff left to see what he could find to give me some relief. I was surprised because I didn't feel this at all when I was running. I had no idea my skin was damaged until I stepped into the shower. Another great example of how hurt and harm didn't always match up. I had injured my skin but had no idea until I got into the shower.

This was just one of the many side effects of running marathons—soreness, discomfort, chafing, grins from ear to ear, pure joy, and did I mention soreness? Oddly, I was already thinking about the next marathon to sign up for. *This is the strange thing about us runners, isn't it?*

Jeff came to my rescue with some cream my aunt had. I slathered it on with several groans and grimaces. *Good Lord, this hurts worse than giving birth.* I managed to get dressed whispering, *Thank you body and thank you mind for another marathon finish.* I grabbed Jeff's hand and I hobbled to the elevators. *Let's eat.*

The restaurant was right by the finish line. I ducked out again to cheer for the runners' finishing. I was so thrilled for everyone crossing the finish. We all did something hard and amazing today. I walked into the restaurant and a waiter approached me. He saw the medal around my neck "Great job! What can I get you to drink?"

"Water would be great!" He handed me water with ice and congratulated me again. He asked how I did and I smiled, "I finished."

The restaurant was two stories with enormous windows to look out at the finish line. I climbed the wooden stairs to meet my family and was overcome with applause. A family had a huge table next to the stairs and saw me coming with my medal on. They were clapping and congratulating me! I couldn't believe it. *Me?* I was so overcome with emotion and couldn't stop thanking them. What a wonderful gesture. They were celebrating too and when I saw runners with medals on, I congratulated them. They were all crowded to-gether watching the race from the window. It was fantastic.

Jeff and I spotted the rest of our family at the table and headed over to join them. I couldn't wait to eat! We gathered around the table and I felt like we were sitting at the finish line. We could hear the announcer calling people's names as they crossed the line. There was a TV in front of us broadcasting the race. Goosebumps covered my arms as I watched the screen. It was cool to learn that Shalane Flanagan was there running as well as Danika Patrick. It was incredible knowing I ran with these famous women. We ordered our food and I began to share the story about the bus getting lost and our adventure to the start line. We laughed, ate, and talked. It was fun to hear my children's side of things and what they did all morning while I was running.

Delaney spoke up first, "We went to breakfast. I ordered french toast and it was huge with lots of butter."

Brindsley chimed in, "I got the same thing, it was so good."

Jeff smiled. Jeff and my mom said they were able to see the entire race from the para-athletes and wheelchair racers, to the top professional men and women finishers. They were amazed.

Brindsley said again, "I want to run The Boston Marathon when I get older."

I smiled, "I would love to run it with you Brindsley."

We finished our meal and headed back outside toward the finish line. Crowds of people still gathered as runners crossed the finish. We cheered and congratulated runners as we passed. I was tired and ready to put my feet up and reflect on the day.

I did it. I finally ran The Boston Marathon, and when I look down at my medal, I'm full of joy.

***

When we got back up to our hotel room, Delaney handed me a handwritten note with a smile on her face. It was written on the hotel paper she found in our room. "LENOX Hotel" was printed on the top. It was perfect. She watched me as I read it trying to hold back tears. She wrote in her best cursive writing:

"I love mom. Congratulations! You did it. Deep inside you have courage! You are the best."

She even added some hearts and stars to decorate the tiny square paper. I bent down and gave her a huge hug and kiss. What a gift it was to be her mother.

Is it just me or do you find yourself crying over the simplest things? Is it motherhood? Is it getting older? Is it love?

This handwritten note was love from my daughter to me. I was overwhelmed with gratitude. My family has supported me day in and day out as I trained to get to this moment. They heard me talk about Boston, read and write about Boston, and watch Boston. I laughed and cried when I finished reading her note. She knew. I didn't think what I was doing had any impact on my family yet it did. My children were watching me, they noticed, and I was showing them the hard work and the joy of running.

Chapter Twenty-Two
Boston Marathon Finisher

My eyes fixed on the pen
My hand hesitant
Body heavy in the chair.
Write something, anything.
I pause—images float to the surface of my mind
I want to shove them back down—forget
Pick up the pen and face yourself, cheers Natalie Goldberg.
I clutch the pen.
My hand begins from left to right
Words appear—memories
printed along the 45 miles of nerves making up my body.
Tingles, burns, and zaps shout in protection.
Keep writing, keep writing.
My pen moves fast across the page
Words not allowed to be said
Truth swept under the rug
in black ink stares back at me.
Keep going, keep going
I hear the whisper from the page
My fist loosens around the pen
I breathe—notice the tension in my back,
hip and shoulders begin to soften.

Inhale, exhale— breath deepens.
My vigilant nervous system is standing down.
My heart slows—no longer racing in fear.
There is no lion here.
Keep writing, keep writing is all I hear.
My back releases its grip with each word safe
to slump over the page — I am safe.
The sentences move down the paper—to confront,
to heal.
I have the right to write, says Julia Cameron.
My shoulders drop from my ears at the last sentence.
I set down the pen until tomorrow
To start again— confront my fears,
write my story, find my voice,
And start again.

I tossed and turned all night. My hips and legs were sore. I was a side sleeper and couldn't get comfortable. My hips ached, and my nerves buzzed with excitement at what I had accomplished.

I shifted onto my back, eyes still closed.

Julie, breathe, relax, sleep.

My mind, however, wanted to recall every minute of what happened today from the adventure of the bus ride, and the lengthy warm-up to the Scream Tunnel and Heartbreak

Hill. I wanted to remember the spectators' cheers, the volunteers, my family who came to support me, and the congratulations from the hotel staff as I made my way into the lobby all while the medal hung around my neck. I wanted to remember every detail, every second. I didn't want to forget a thing and found myself repeating as much as I could over and over.

I finally ran Boston, I did it. I couldn't sleep. I wanted to run through the streets and celebrate! My eyes opened. I was wide awake.

I knew sleep would help my recovery yet I just couldn't settle down so I decided to get up. I couldn't lie here another minute. I decided to go down to the lobby to grab a cup of coffee and go for a walk. I also needed to write down what was swirling in my mind. I had so many words that needed to come out. I slipped out of bed making sure not to wake my family. I tiptoed to the bathroom to throw on some clothes, grabbed my bag, and put my notebook and pen inside. I headed towards the lobby hoping the sound of the door clicking shut didn't wake Jeff and the kids.

I crept down the hallway to the elevator. *Oh, shoot, where is my mask?* I reached into my sweatshirt praying I still had the one from yesterday. I didn't want to head back to the room. *Oh good, it's still here.* I placed it around my nose and mouth as I made my way into the elevator. No one else joined me. I wondered if other runners were having trouble sleeping.

The elevator doors opened and I was greeted by the coffee aroma wafting through the lobby. My nose nudged me over to grab a cup before heading outside. The dark hot liquid circled the cup warming my hands. I popped a lid on and headed out to the city streets. I forgot how bright it would be even at this hour.

Walking after a marathon was great for recovery and since I couldn't sleep, this was my next best option. I figured it would be quiet on the streets just like in the hotel but I was surprised to see other runners doing the same as me—taking a walk. I guess I wasn't the only one who couldn't sleep. Perhaps they were soaking in what they had just accomplished and walking off their soreness too.

Clang. Bang. Where was that noise coming from? I looked to the right to see the finish line set up starting to come down. Several men were already working on taking everything apart. It was bittersweet. The Boston Marathon was over.

I stood on the sidewalk watching the men work for a moment as I sipped my coffee. A few runners were getting pictures of the paintings on the street that were smudged and worn from all the foot traffic yesterday. I turned towards the public gardens. *I'll walk 15 minutes out then turn around and come back.* The noise of the workers started to fade as I headed towards Charles Street where the buses lined up yesterday to take us to the start line. The start area that I didn't get to experience would be my motivation to get back here again. I didn't want to miss a thing about this marathon and I felt that I had missed something at the starting line. I couldn't help but wonder, *were there tents up and volunteers whom I didn't get to see and thank? Where exactly did the buses drop everyone off? What was the atmosphere like? Was there music playing and runners hanging out before they made their walk to the start?* I didn't know. I wasn't there. I had a different start and one I was choosing to be grateful for. I noticed managing my mind, pivoting and adapting when things didn't go as planned, controlling my emotions, and redirecting my thoughts were improving. I was glad it happened. I was proud of myself for responding the way I did and for not letting negative thoughts consume my mind or change my attitude.

Paying attention to my thoughts mattered. Motherhood and running were helping me practice this daily. *I am valuable and resilient.*

I looked down at my watch. Fifteen minutes had already passed. I turned around and walked back toward where all the excitement took place yesterday—seeing my family cheering for me, meeting other runners, and the volunteers and medical staff helping us all at the finish. What an amazing day. I recalled meeting Stephanie. What a blessing and joy it was to meet her. She was someone I felt I already knew. I wanted to ask her if we had met before even though I knew we hadn't.

The city was rather still as I stood at the corner of Boylston and Exeter Street sipping my coffee. My mind flashed images of what I experienced from the entire start to finish. I had run eight other marathons yet, this one was different.

Is it because it's been my dream for so long and I've had to pivot many times to get here? Is it Boston, the history, or the prestige of this marathon that makes this so special?

I suppose it was all of this. I finally accomplished my mission.

I closed my eyes, soaking in the memory. I wanted to savor every moment and take time to celebrate even if it was alone on Boylston street. It felt great to take in the morning air and honor what I had accomplished. A journey that took so much of my life was now over. I did it. What a bittersweet feeling. I've been chasing after this dream for so long—*What now? What will be your goal now?* I would celebrate this achievement and would answer that question when I returned home.

***

My family and I stayed for a few more days to enjoy the sights. As we headed out of the hotel that Tuesday morning, I saw an enormous line down Boylston Street coming from the Marathon Sports running store. *Huh, I wonder what's going on there?* A runner with a medal around her neck passed me and I asked if she knew. "Oh, yes I'm going there right now. They're engraving our medals with your time and name."

"Oh great. Thank you and congratulations!"

"You too!" I didn't have my medal with me so I told Jeff that I'd go there after lunch. We were headed to the Duck Tours and I didn't want to change our plans. (The Duck Tours was fantastic by the way, I highly recommend it.)

My family and I were enjoying the sights when perfect strangers would come up to me, and congratulate me. I was delighted to be greeted by so many people all because of a foot race. They asked, "How did you do?" or "How did the race go?" *How did they know?* I guess it was the Boston Marathon apparel I had on or was it the glow that so many runners talked about? Each encounter brought smiles, laughter, and excitement. I walked away from each meeting full of joy.

After lunch, I headed over to the store to find out how much longer they would be engraving medals. The man looked down at his watch, then at me, "Three more minutes." I thought he was joking but he wasn't.

"I'm going to get my medal right now, I'll be right back."

I dashed ahead of Jeff, " I'll meet you back at the hotel after I get my medal engraved."

I took off running, my legs forgetting that I just ran a marathon yesterday. *I hope they wait for me.* I hurried into the hotel and stood by the elevator. It was taking too long so I took the stairs. The stairs were the last thing I wanted to climb but I wanted my medal engraved. I made a mad dash down the hall to our room, grabbed my medal on the coffee table, and headed back to the stairs. I didn't want to waste time waiting for the elevator. I hobbled down the stairs with my medal in hand. *Please still be there.* I rushed out of the hotel and back down Boylston Street just in time. I made it and was grateful they waited for me.

***

Two days after finishing The Boston Marathon I was still having a hard time sleeping. I was lying on my back looking up at the hotel ceiling. I heard a few sirens outside our window. Brindsley was next to me sound asleep. My chatter started. *Could I have run faster? Why did I have such a hard time pacing this course?* I was disappointed I didn't qualify for Boston again. I wanted to be back here in April. *I forgot to get gifts for my family. Maybe I didn't take in enough hydration early on. No, it was probably because of that two-mile walk.*

My mind was racing. My thoughts jumped around from one thing to another. Of course, I couldn't sleep with all the ruckus in my mind. *Julie, what are you going to do?* Oh, it's Aunt Phoebe, again. I'd spent the last ten years learning to be aware of the mindless chatter that keeps me in doubt, fear, and worries.

It was getting easier to notice and be aware of the negative thoughts but I didn't sleep well the two nights in Boston after the race. I promised myself I wouldn't do this but here I was beating myself up again and second-guessing my performance. I listened to the negative self-talk and my mind raced with the "should've" and "could've." *You didn't even have the pain you normally have. Why didn't you run faster? You didn't run fast enough to qualify for Boston.* I let those thoughts get the best of me. After two nights of no sleep, I reached out to Joel. My coach was someone I felt safe talking to. I shared with him the thoughts that were coming up and my trouble with sleep.

He texted me, "It's normal to reflect and question. This has been a journey and just because you've crossed the finish line doesn't necessarily mean it's over."

I let him know that I was beating myself up because I didn't have the hip pain or any nerve-related symptoms which I'd experienced at every marathon race since 2011. I was waiting for the pain to show up at mile 14 but it never did! I was surprised and happy yet the race was over and I was questioning my performance. *I should've run faster.* I didn't have the nerve pain to deal with though I was dealing with the other parts of the marathon. Staying hydrated, fighting off a cramp in my quadricep and hamstring, and fatigue from the hills but I had no nerve symptoms in my hip or leg which I'd grown accustomed to. It was incredible to run without those symptoms.

He responded, "No pain or nerve-related symptoms are HUGE!! That's a success in and of itself. Boston is a tough course and pacing is a challenge to nail on your first attempt. Considering the conditions, first time on the course, etc. I think you had a great race!"

I was so glad I shared with Joel what was on my mind. I felt better after letting him know what I was struggling with. The next night, I slept great. I laughed. Why didn't I reach out to him sooner? It was a good reminder for me. *It's okay to ask for help. It's important to share what's on my mind with someone I feel safe with if it's affecting my sleep and mood.*

Chapter Twenty-Three
What Now?

Rolling over rocks
Finds a way around the bend
Pushing through the leaves
Gentle, yet mighty
Keeps flowing— continues on
Be the stream, bounce on!

We pulled into the driveway. We had made it home. I peered through the driver's side window and saw balloons and a huge poster board set up outside our home. The balloons were tied to the chair just outside our garage. *Oh my gosh! What is that?*

Jeff parked the car and I hurried out to see the amazing setup. The balloons read, "Congratulations! Way to go! Amazing!" The poster board was decorated with bright colors and stickers congratulating me on my finish in Boston. *Wow, who is this from?* My mind wondered who would come up with such a generous idea. I saw a bright blue envelope. It was from my friend, Toni.

Brindsley and Delaney began tossing the balloons around and I sat on the floor in front of the poster board reading the words, "You did it!" "Julie, you are amazing!" "Hooray, Boom," and "So happy for you." I was stunned. What a wonderful surprise and gift. It made my day and I couldn't thank her enough for her kindness and generosity.

The glow that I'd been carrying since I finished The Boston Marathon was even brighter. The love and support from my family and friends had been more than I could imagine. I opened my email to find cheer cards from friends, family, and running buddies. I checked in with my text messages and made sure to text everyone back. I felt loved and I was so happy to be home to continue celebrating this long-awaited goal. I couldn't wait to connect with friends and family to tell them all about it.

***

I wanted to get back to Boston. I was disappointed that I didn't qualify again when I was there. Maybe I could still qualify. *I wonder if there is another local marathon I can do before the end of the year.* This was my adrenaline and runner's high talking, still running the show a week after Boston. I got on the computer and searched for marathons in New York. New York City was in November yet that wasn't something I could register for. Then I saw a marathon in Syracuse, New York (15 minutes from my home) in one week. *Hmm, I could run that.* I was feeling good. I could run another marathon in a week. I texted my coach and shared with him my crazy idea. Luckily, he calmly responded, "That's too soon."

Shalane Flanagan was doing it, why can't I? My coach talked me down from the cloud I was on. "We didn't plan this or set up your training for this. Rest and recover. You will get back here, and I want you to get back here."

I was glad he brought me back down to reality—saving me from myself. Prioritizing sleep, nutrition, and active recovery was what I needed to focus on this next month and Joel reminded me of this. He was right. I would get back here and the best part was it wouldn't take me 20 years this time.

I went out for my first run five days after Boston. I was sore. I was crazy to think I could run another marathon a week later. Sure I probably could push through 26.2 miles but to qualify for Boston was pushing it. My legs ached and it was an effort to keep placing one foot in front of the other. Of course, when I saw a woman like Shalane Flanagan racing six marathons in six weeks, I thought I should be able to do that too. The difference was she had a plan. I did not. I was going purely off emotion and probably a little ego. The awesome thing was to have women runners going for it and taking on huge goals. It was inspiring.

***

It was hard to believe that it was a week ago that I ran The Boston Marathon. I was still glowing and wanted to slow down and enjoy this achievement a little bit longer. So many times in my life I achieved a goal then it was right on to the next thing—no time for celebration or reflection. I wanted it to be different this time. I wanted to savor this accomplishment. I didn't want to rush right into the next thing.

This wasn't easy. Yet I wanted to soak it in for a while and be proud, happy, and grateful for what my body and mind accomplished. This was a dream that I hung onto for so long. I couldn't put into words everything I was feeling. It was tremendous. God's timing was perfect. Yet, when I couldn't run The Boston Marathon in 2003, I was angry, disappointed, and frustrated. Yet God knows what is best for us. His love never fails. He is always faithful. It's incredible for me to think about. He answered my prayers—in his perfect timing. The challenges and troubles I faced led me to this victorious day.

***

What now? I asked that question again. What about running an Ultramarathon? A new challenge and distance, a goal to focus on next.

It was after the Fargo Marathon in 2017 that I began thinking about running Ultras. I was staying at a hotel in Fargo when I met Dan. He was from Canada and was there with his buddies running the marathon too. We started talking over coffee in the lobby. He shared with me the races he had done. He started talking about Ultra distances. I was amazed and inspired to hear his stories. The excitement he had when sharing his experiences was contagious. I wanted to experience his energy too. He was encouraging, smiling at me "You would love it."

Dan's eyes lit up as he continued to share with me all the ultras he and his buddies have done. As we talked, I felt he was someone I met before like we were old friends. I loved when this happened. I find it easy to be myself.

I was noticing this more when I met people. It was a feeling I cherished and one I was not taking for granted. I believe it was God's way of telling me that it is okay for me to be myself. I didn't have to apologize anymore for being me. I was worthy and lovable. I was someone to get to know. I could open myself up to other people and experiences.

For many years of my life, I closed myself off because of fear. Fear of not being good enough, fear of saying the wrong thing, and fear of I wasn't worthy. *Who wants to talk to me? Who would want to get to know me?* Well, in these years of pursuing my dream, I learned it was a lie. I was missing out on my life, and I wasn't sharing my gifts with the world.

When I got home from Fargo, I purchased a book, "Running Your First Ultra" by Krissy Moehl. I looked through it and imagined running 50 miles in the future. I decided after I raced The Boston Marathon I was going to run an Ultra. I said that to myself though with hesitation. At the time, I was diagnosed with psoriatic arthritis, and there was plenty of doubt that it wasn't in the cards for me. Yet, my diagnosis was not my destiny, something I was repeating to myself as I was training and researching. I tucked the thought away and placed the book in the cabinet. It would have to wait. My focus was on Boston and I wanted to achieve my dream before I thought about anything else. The idea of running an ultra didn't seem so crazy to me. I loved to run and the longer I ran the better I felt. Diagnosis or not, I knew it would be my next goal after Boston.

***

When I got home from The Boston Marathon the thought I'm going to run an Ultra reemerged. *Oh yes, I remember now.* I opened the cabinet where I had tucked the book away. I pulled it out and smiled. I was going to run an ultra in 2022. I began researching races close to home and what would work for my racing plan. I talked with Joel and let him know what I was thinking. He was onboard and thought I would do well in an ultra race. I was happy he would be willing to coach me as well. We planned the racing calendar for 2022 with a half marathon in March, a marathon in April (yes I do want to get back to Boston), and a 50-mile ultra in September. It felt good to have race goals in place. I needed goals to keep going on the days or weeks life got messy. It kept me focused and optimistic.

I shared these goals with my family and they were all for me getting back to Boston. My husband couldn't believe how amazing it was. He wasn't a runner so for him to be as excited as I was, well it was incredible! I was blessed to have my family's support.

Epilogue

Brindsley and me heading out the door
This morning run will not be a bore
Our laughter fills the quiet roads
The grin across my face shows
Joy in running with my son
Time together is so much fun!
The fall colors all around
Crunching leaves on the ground

Legs getting tired, and a side stitch
slows us down. But we won't quit
We'll walk for a bit.
We got each other to make the climb
In running and life, we'll make the time
To slow down and enjoy the pace—
slow down and see each other's face
Brindsley I love you
You're my sunshine and grace

Brindsley and I were the first ones up. I had an easy 35-minute run planned and I asked Brindsley if he wanted to run with me. I was so happy he said yes. I needed his energy and smile to get out the door. We headed toward the village. His chatter and laughter energized me the entire run. He kept talking about Boston and how his dream was now to run the Boston Marathon. I again told him I hope to run it with him.

He said he loves to run, "Wouldn't it be great if I won it, mom?"

I grinned, "Yes it would!"

Then he said, "I don't think I would want to be interviewed though."

He made me laugh. I loved his questions and his marvelous thinking. We continued running in silence then he spoke up about a girl in his class. He told me he had a crush on her.

"Mom, how do I get her to notice me? We aren't in the same class."

"Well maybe just start with a smile or a wave when you see her." I was so happy he felt comfortable talking to me and grateful for the time with him on the road. He was learning, just like me, how the road holds space for us. *When we have a buddy to run with it's a time to let go of our worries and set them down on the road. Mile after mile, let it go.*

Thank you body for another awesome training run today. Thank you body for another race. I say this often and after every run. And more importantly, I believe it. The joy that I found as a child has returned and the pressure to please and perform well, I've let go. I no longer need to carry that burden. I run for myself and the joy it brings. I run for writing, connecting with nature, feeling God's presence, dreaming, and thinking about what I want to be when I grow up.

The belief that I would run Boston—even during the setbacks, troubles, and challenges—was my mission. It was on this journey toward Boston that I faced myself, challenged my default stories, and strengthened my relationship with God. What I discovered and learned about fighting for this dream was self-love, forgiveness, and God's faithfulness. In the pain and struggle came growth, newfound gratitude, and appreciation. This process allowed me to show up for my children. It wouldn't have been possible if I didn't have a dream I was pursuing—if I didn't have the gift of running in my life. The gift the good Lord gave me.

A Reading List

A few books that have inspired and guided me
(in no particular order)

Essential Sports Nutrition: A Guide to Optimal Performance for Every Active Person by Marni Sumbal, MS, RD, CSSD, LD/N

ROAR by Stacy T. Sims, PhD

The Boston Marathon: The History of the World's Premier Running Event by Tom Derderian

Let Your Mind Run, A Memoir of Thinking My Way to Victory by Deena Kastor and Michelle Hamilton

Finding Your Sweet Spot: How to Avoid RED-S by optimizing Your Energy Balance by Rebecca McConville, MS RD CSSD CEDRD

Run Fast. Eat Slow. Nourishing Recipes for Athletes by Shalane Flanagan & Elyse Kopecky

Run Fast. Cook Fast. Eat Slow. by Shalane Flanagan & Elyse Kopecky

Rise & Run. by Shalane Flanagan & Elyse Kopecky

How Bad do You Want It? By Matt Fitzgerald

Run to Overcome by Meb Keflezighi

Meb for Mortals by Meb Keflezighi

26 Marathons by Meb Keflezighi

This is The Day: Reclaim Your Dream. Ignite Your Passion. Live your Purpose by Tim Tebow

The Champion Mindset: An Athlete's Guide To Mental Toughness by Joanna Zeiger, Ph.D.

The Long Run: A NYC Firefighter's Triumphant Comeback From Crash Victim To Elite Athlete by Matt Long with Charles Butler

Get Out Of Your Head: Stopping the Spiral of Toxic Thoughts by Jennie Allen

The Art of Possibility by Rosamund Stone Zander and Benjamin Zander

Endure: Mind, Body, and the Curiously Elastic Limits of Human Performance by Alex Hutchinson

Thrive by Brendan Brazier

Uncommon Heart by Anne Audain and John L. Parker, Jr.

Good For a Girl by Lauren Fleshman

Mental Training for Ultrarunning by Addie Bracy

Running Your First Ultra by Krissy Moehl

Finding Ultra: Rejecting Middle Age, Becoming One of the World's Fittest Men, and Discovering Myself by Rich Roll

The Obstacle Is the Way by Ryan Holiday

Gratitudes

I am overcome with gratitude as I recall all the people who have helped me during the writing of this book. It really does take a village.

First my amazing children, Brindsley and Delaney. My one rule in the morning has been *don't come out of your room until 6:30 am.* (This allowed me the opportunity to run and write before mother duties began.) Thank you for honoring "mom time". I'm so blessed to be your mama. Thank you for your amazing patience with me and I pray this book encourages you to never stop dreaming.

Jeff thank you for your support not only in running but writing. Thank you for giving me the space to do both things I truly love—alone. I'm grateful to be doing life with you. *Let's get back to Boston!* I love you.

Many thanks to Joel Sattgast, my friend and coach, I wouldn't have toed the start line without you. Thank you for believing in me. Your can-do attitude, wisdom, knowledge, and "you will make it" was just what I needed. Thank you for being a consistent person in my corner. This book is my way of paying it forward.

Thank you to Marni Sumbal, you are a blessing. I don't want to even think about where I would be without your guidance, wisdom, kindness, and knowledge. Working with you sparked a change in me and I was ready—thank you! Your book lives in my kitchen so when those old thoughts creep in about carbohydrates I open your book and read your words to get back on track. It's a constant reminder of how far I've come and to continue down the path of healthy choices. Thank you. I'm so happy our paths crossed and I have Christopher Johnson to thank.

Thank you, Christopher Johson, it was through your Runner's Zone Facebook group that I had the opportunity to meet Joel and Marni. Your knowledge, generosity, consistent value, and resources challenged my thinking and guided me down a path of tremendous growth and curiosity. Your willingness to show up will never be forgotten. I'm so grateful our paths have crossed. I am running healthy, happy, and strong because of you, Joel, and Marni. I feel privileged to have been offered your expertise and wisdom.

To my Beta Readers: Karen Bloom, Felicia Case, Jeanne Cioci, and Cathy Hughes thank you for taking the time to read and share your input. I appreciate your support, encouragement, and thoughts to make this book better.

I would like to thank Penny Brucker for editing and formatting this manuscript. Thank you for working so diligently to meet my deadline. I appreciate your thoughtful feedback and patience.

A huge thank you to Writing in Community (WIC)— I'm thrilled I found this community to push my writing into practice and ship imperfect work daily. It was through this practice of showing up that my book was created. I must thank— Terri Tomoff, Bill Tomoff, Kymberly Dakin, Heather Button, Julie Rains, Linda McLachlan, Pierre Powell, Linda Platt, Kathy Taylor, Kathy Karn, Diane Osgood, Michal Berman, Ame Sanders, Carolina Perez, Louise Karch, Kristin Hatcher, Seth Godin, Cindy Villanueva, Amanda Hsiung-Blodgett, Russell John, Kristi Casey, Kerry Itami, Melissa Kalinowski, Laurie Riedman, Joyce Sullivan, Benjamin Boekweg, Trent Selbrede, Susan Fritz, Deborah Mourey—to have you alongside me each day, especially on the days my inner judge would creep in, was powerful. It was knowing I had you cheering me on that kept me going. Thank you for being a safe space to do that. I had no idea the impact it would have on me and my family. My children are writing books now! Thank you for your support, encouragement, wisdom, inspiration, and above all your kindness and generosity. I'm truly blessed to know each of you and I'm still amazed at the outpouring of love you've shown me. I am sincerely grateful our paths have crossed and I hope we continue to write together. Onward!

To my friends on Facebook, thank you for taking the time to share my message with others. It's been a joy to have help when I'm not the best at asking for help. Thank you for knowing this and taking it upon yourself to spread the word. I'm learning this is a process and help is a blessing. Thank you, Mom, Cathy Hughes, Felicia Case, Cindy Myderk, Jeanne Cioci, Terri Tomoff, Aunt Colleen Bloom, and Jennifer Harvey.

To the Run to Write Community, thank you for supporting my work and meeting up on Fridays to write together. It's been a pleasure to get to know you— Holly Rabalais, Sharon Shimpach, Rebecca Holden, Amie McGraham, Melissa Mapstone, Beth Wild, and Camille Prairie. I look forward to our meet-ups each week.

Stephanie Key— my Boston run buddy! You are a joy and I'm thrilled we met at our first Boston Marathon. I'm still glowing. Thank you for allowing me to share our conversation in this book and our picture. You are awesome and I will never forget your kindness. I truly feel like we have met before. I hope to see you soon. Happy running.

Thank you to Toni Carrington for being you! What an amazing welcome home surprise you delivered. Thank you for your generosity and encouragement. You really know how to make a person feel special. Thanks a million.

Thank you to Karen Bloom, for your support and love. I can't thank you enough for making the trip to Boston and helping Jeff and me with Brindsley and Delaney. It made us feel lighter knowing you were there and to have an extra set of hands in a big city. Thank you for your endless support these last 42 years!

To my siblings, Jon Bloom, Mandy Rundgren, Michelle Ball, and Becky Stanford, thank you for the text messages and the cheer cards. It made my day knowing you were cheering me on from afar.

Thank you to Mike Bloom and Sally Dulcich-Bloom for the message and congratulations! It was wonderful to know that you cared.

Many thanks to Colleen and Tim Bloom, Jed and Arunima Bloom, and Family, and Jeremy Bloom—thank you for making the trip to Boston to support and cheer me on. It was awesome to have you there to share this long-awaited dream. The cheer poster was awesome and it made my day.

A million thanks to Carrie-Anne Haag, Felicia Case, and Jeanne Cioci for your support in so many generous ways as I worked on this book. Your friendship is a gift. Thank you.

I'm grateful to the local running community, Fleet Feet, and especially the race directors Rick Streeter, Deb Cerelli, and Roxanne Carrier for the opportunity to hang out at your incredible race events and share my books. Thank you.

Finally—Thank you, God. It is through You that this book is possible. Thank you, Lord, for giving me the gifts to share my story with others. May the words in this book speak to their heart and may it bless their life in the way You have intended.

Stay in Touch

Subscribe to Run to Write, *Transforming runs to words one poem at a time:* juliebhughes.substack.com

Listen in: Run to Write Poetry Podcast— on Apple Podcasts or Spotify

Email: hughesjulie413@gmail.com

Facebook: www.facebook.com/juliebhughes

About the Author

Julie B. Hughes is a licensed physical therapist who loves to run, write, cook, hike, and be outdoors. She lives in Manlius, NY with her husband and two children. She is grateful for her running and the joy it brings her. You can find her weekday blog, Run to Write at juliebhughes.substack.com.

More from Julie B. Hughes

My Road: A Runner's Journey Through Persistent Pain to Healing

Run to Boston: Poems for the Marathoner

Running Into Poetry: An invitation to be present on your path

Email me if you would like a copy:
hughesjulie413@gmail.com

Or they can be found on Amazon.

Made in the USA
Columbia, SC
03 March 2023

13264029R00117